TRANSNATIONAL REPRODUCTION

ANTHROPOLOGIES OF AMERICAN MEDICINE:
CULTURE, POWER, AND PRACTICE

General Editors: Paul Brodwin, Michele Rivkin-Fish, and Susan Shaw

Transnational Reproduction: Race, Kinship,
and Commercial Surrogacy in India
Daisy Deomampo

Transnational Reproduction

Race, Kinship, and Commercial Surrogacy in India

Daisy Deomampo

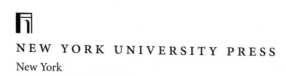

NEW YORK UNIVERSITY PRESS
New York

NEW YORK UNIVERSITY PRESS
New York
www.nyupress.org

References to Internet websites (URLs) were accurate at the time of writing. Neither the author nor New York University Press is responsible for URLs that may have expired or changed since the manuscript was prepared.

ISBN: 978-1-4798-0421-4 (hardback)
ISBN: 978-1-4798-2838-8 (paperback)

For Library of Congress Cataloging-in-Publication data, please contact the Library of Congress.

New York University Press books are printed on acid-free paper, and their binding materials are chosen for strength and durability. We strive to use environmentally responsible suppliers and materials to the greatest extent possible in publishing our books.

Manufactured in the United States of America

10 9 8 7 6 5 4 3 2 1

Also available as an ebook

To my parents,

Fe and Dominador Deomampo

CONTENTS

ACKNOWLEDGMENTS

First and foremost, this book would not have been possible without the generosity and kindness of those who invited me into their homes and lives in the course of this research. I have changed names and personal information to protect privacy, and I regret that I cannot express my thanks to everyone by name. I am grateful to the Indian women I met who were or wanted to become surrogate mothers and egg donors—thank you for telling me your stories and for transforming the way I see the world. I am especially thankful to the woman I call Antara. Antara welcomed me into her home, fed me delicious meals, and understood the importance of this research from the very start; without her I would never have met many of the surrogate mothers and egg donors whose stories grace this book. I also extend my gratitude to the intended parents and parents of children born through surrogacy in India. I am thankful they shared their time and experiences with me, amidst stressful stays in India and busy lives with small children. I also thank the doctors, lawyers, medical tourism agents and brokers, and U.S. Consulate General staff in Mumbai for taking time out from their busy schedules to assist me in my fieldwork.

Although I studied Hindi before beginning fieldwork, I required the assistance of translators for my interviews with surrogates and egg donors (who spoke mainly Marathi and Hindi). Thus, I am greatly indebted to my research assistants, Prachi Bari, Kaveri Dadhich, Vasudha Mohanka, and Mrinmayee Ranade; they proved to be skilled translators as well as astute observers, and I am grateful for their insights and service. Prachi, who worked with me in the majority of interviews with surrogate mothers, deserves special thanks for her enthusiasm for this project, willingness to travel long distances, and tireless energy even amid long days of interviews. I thank Abby Rabinowitz and Kainaz Amaria for keeping me sane during fieldwork. I owe profound thanks to Abby, who was working on her own surrogacy project in India when we met and who introduced me to several key participants in this research. Fieldwork in Mumbai would have been far less rich, interesting, and enjoyable without her. Thank you to the wonderful staff at the Tata Institute of Social Sciences who welcomed me as a visiting research scholar during my fieldwork in 2010.

I am deeply grateful to Leith Mullings, Katherine Verdery, Murphy Halliburton, and Rayna Rapp for providing invaluable comments, advice, and support. Thank you also to fellow writing group members for your enthusiasm for this project and for always challenging me to think about this work in new ways: Ujju Aggarwal, Sophie Bjork-James, Maggie Dickinson, Harmony Goldberg, Andrea Morrell, and Karen G. Williams.

So many people offered encouragement and support at key junctures along the way; crucially, they gave advice on research strategies when I needed it, commented on conference papers and chapter drafts, and were welcome interlocutors on all topics related to surrogacy and assisted reproduction in India: Aditya Bharadwaj, Risa Cromer, Bishakha Datta, Rebecca Haimowitz, Marcia Inhorn, Amar Jesani, David Kertzer, Martha Lincoln, Lakshmi Lingam, Anindita Majumdar, Purnima Mankekar, Lauren Jade Martin, Sarojini N., Vimla Nadkarni, Sharmila Rudrappa, Chayanika Shah, Molly Shanley, Nayantara Sheoran, Holly Donahue Singh, Vaishali Sinha, Sandhya Srinivasan, Elly Teman, and Cecilia Van Hollen. I must also thank colleagues at the 2011 and 2012 Tarrytown Meetings, as well as the 2014 International Forum on Intercountry Adoption and Global Surrogacy at the International Institute of Social Studies in The Hague. Conversations at these meetings pushed me to think about the social and ethical implications of my research in critical ways; my sincerest thanks to Marcy Darnovsky at the Center for Genetics and Society for inviting me to attend these meetings and for her ongoing support of my work. Wholehearted thanks to my current colleagues at Fordham University, especially Orit Avishai, Hugo Benavides, Evelyn Bush, Ayala Fader, Jeanne Flavin, Christine Fountain, Allan Gilbert, Micki McGee, Aseel Sawalha, and Matthew Weinshenker, who offered generous camaraderie and advice on all things teaching and research related. I am lucky to have landed at such a welcoming place at the start of my career.

Multiple institutions provided the financial support and time necessary for completing this book. They include the Foreign Language and Area Studies (FLAS) Fellowship from the University of Wisconsin, research grants from the National Science Foundation and the Wenner-Gren Foundation, writing fellowships from the Ford Foundation and the City University of New York, a faculty research grant from Fordham University, and the Hunt Postdoctoral Fellowship from the Wenner-Gren Foundation. Portions of this book appear in the journals *Medical Anthropology*, *Frontiers: A Journal of Women's Studies*, and *positions: asia critique*. An earlier draft of chapter 3 benefited immensely from comments at the Workshop on Intimate Industries in Asia at Pomona College; thank you to fellow participants as well as to the organizers, Rhacel Salazar Parreñas, Hung Cam Thai, and Rachel Silvey, and especially to Rhacel for inviting me to participate. I presented an earlier version of chapter 6 at the Conference on Population and Development: Anthropological Perspectives at Brown University; I thank the organizers, Daniel Jordan Smith and Jennifer Johnson-Hanks, as well as fellow participants for their generous feedback. I owe profound thanks to Jennifer Hammer at NYU Press for her enthusiasm and support of this project, as well as to the anonymous reviewers whose comments greatly improved the arguments set forth in this book. I must also acknowledge the fine editorial work of Kate Epstein, without whom this book would have been far less readable.

Lastly, I must thank my family and friends who have encouraged and sustained me, and tolerated endless chatter about surrogacy in India over the years: Jude, Joseph, Julie, Susan, Jesse, Daniel, Aimee, Erin, Sarah, Saralé, Melissa, and of course my extended Lorenzo family in LA. Heartfelt thanks to Sheila and Isaac Heimbinder for being the most supportive and generous parents-in-law one could ask for; and thank you to Isaac for tirelessly e-mailing news stories and sending clippings over the years. My deepest gratitude to my parents, Fe and Dominador Deomampo, whose own journeys from the Philippines have inspired my enduring interests in globalization, inequality, and social justice. I thank them for their unconditional love and support (even when I followed a sometimes perplexing and winding career path). I regret that I could not share this book with my late father and father-in-law; my father's kindness and care and my father-in-law's curiosity and interest nurtured me throughout the years it took to complete this work. Finally, to my husband, Michael, whom I cannot thank enough for his intellectual engagement and practical support; from reading multiple drafts to providing childcare, I could not have written this book without him. And to our children, Mirabelle and Lorenzo, who have enriched my life beyond measure.

Introduction

On a Sunday afternoon in the midst of monsoon season, I sat in a hotel restaurant sipping coffee with Eben,[1] a Middle Eastern entrepreneur who had landed in Mumbai several days earlier. Eben's company facilitates surrogacy arrangements in India for prospective parents from all over the world. Eben, whose daughter was born via gestational surrogacy in the United States, explained to me the core motivation for starting his company: to make gestational surrogacy a feasible option for more infertile straight couples and gay couples like him and his male partner. According to Eben, most of his clients simply couldn't afford surrogacy in the United States, and many of them required the assistance of egg donation and preferred a white egg donor who might physically resemble them. Yet surrogacy and egg donation in India seemed daunting; many of Eben's clients were concerned about the quality of medical care and viewed India as a chaotic, poverty-stricken Third World country. Eben thought, pragmatically, "Let's find a way to mix the two [egg donation in the United States and surrogacy in India]." His first clients were a Middle Eastern gay couple; Eben shipped frozen sperm from one of the male partners to the United States, where doctors used it to fertilize donor eggs from a white U.S. woman, then froze and shipped the resulting embryos to India. There, Indian doctors thawed and transferred the embryos into the uterus of an Indian woman.

As Eben went on to explain different aspects of his business, he noted that he does not match clients and surrogates prior to embryo transfer. Instead, doctors transfer embryos into the wombs of surrogates who happen to be prepared to undergo transfer at that time, and the commissioning parents and surrogates sign the contract only after pregnancy is confirmed. In fact, he explained, "Just today I came from a meeting with twelve pregnant surrogates for my clients. We met today and we did all these signatures [for the contracts]." As I imagined Eben in a room filled with a dozen pregnant Indian women, distributing and explaining the contents of the surrogacy contracts, I thought about how this piece of paper, the contract—as well as the fetuses growing inside them—connected the surrogates to parents who lived half a world away and whom they would likely never meet.

Several days later, I was sitting on the floor of Nishi's single-room home in Nadipur,[2] a city located less than forty miles outside Mumbai, snacking on samosas and sipping hot chai. Nishi, a surrogate who was then five months pregnant, proceeded to tell me about her week. She excitedly told me that several days earlier she had discovered where her commissioning parent was from: "My client is Muslim! He is from Dubai, and his name is Omar Chasan." (Surrogates and doctors typically refer to commissioning parents as clients.) When I asked how she knew all this, she explained that she had not actually met Mr. Chasan. In fact, no one had provided her with any information about him, apart from the fact that he was a foreigner. Instead, she told me, she guessed the client's place of origin from the name she read on the contract she had signed earlier that week. She went on to explain, "I didn't meet the client, I met with somebody else who came to get the agreement signed. He was carrying twelve contracts with him and we were twelve surrogates in the room. He took my photograph, asked me my name, and went away." The "guest" pressed a five hundred-rupee bill (approximately U.S.$11)[3] into Nishi's hand, took photographs of Nishi and the other surrogates, and left with the signed contracts.

I had been meeting regularly with Nishi over the past several months, so I was struck by the coincidence when I realized that she must have met Eben on the day she signed the contract—the same day I met with him, one of just a few for which he would be in India. I thought about how Nishi's narrative, like Eben's presence and departure, revealed connections and absences—connections with a "client," the future father of the child she was carrying, who nonetheless remained distinctly absent throughout her pregnancy and, later, recovery from childbirth via cesarean section.

More connections and absences would unfold in various ways in the course of my research. That same week, I met with five white South African women who had traveled to Mumbai as "traveling egg donors," four of whom were returning as second-time egg donors in India. All had donated multiple times in South Africa. They regaled me with their stories of egg donation, shopping, and tourism in India, but also posed thoughtful speculation about the lives of surrogates and intended parents, whom they would never meet. Several months later, I met a Middle Eastern gay couple who had recently become parents to twin girls. I learned they were Eben's clients; a white South African woman had supplied her eggs while an Indian woman provided gestational surrogacy. The couple were curious about the impact that surrogacy had on the lives of surrogate mothers, and lamented that they could not follow up with their surrogate personally, as their doctor strictly forbade any contact.

Throughout my fieldwork, I noted how the lives of surrogates, commissioning parents, egg donors, and brokers converged in Mumbai at distinct moments, sharing a common "quest for conception" (Inhorn 1994). Yet while the process of surrogacy connected these varied actors in far-flung locales, they were effectively absent from each others' everyday lives. The fates of these wide-ranging reproductive actors might intersect in Mumbai at one point or another, but they do not always meet face-to-face, and when they do meet, their interactions are often brief and stilted. Nonetheless, the conception of human life intertwines their lives and they negotiate these connections in ways I didn't expect.

This book is about the ways in which surrogate mothers, parents, egg donors, and agents, among other actors, navigate their relationships formed through gestational surrogacy. It is about race and kinship, and the ways in which transnational reproduction reflects and reinforces local and global inequalities. While commissioning parents, egg donors, surrogates, and doctors come together across transnational and local socioeconomic hierarchies, their understanding of their relationships illuminates how various actors negotiate the intersections of kinship and inequality in transnational contexts. Transnational reproduction commodifies sperm, eggs, and wombs, yet the people I met tended to talk about their interaction as if money had little to do with it. This obscures the power differentials inherent in these processes, and hierarchies of ethnicity, class, gender, and nationality flourish.

Encounters (or the lack thereof) between surrogates and clients shape many of the personal and familial dramas of the people involved in transnational surrogacy. Yet as I began to focus on the relationships between surrogates and clients, I noted the ways in which actors' understandings of kinship and relatedness often relied on naturalized understandings of racialized difference. I began to refine an empirical puzzle that focused on the intersection of race, kinship, and inequality. If transnational surrogacy reinforces global and local stratifications, what are the ideologies of race and kinship that make this possible? How do actors engage racial discourses in order to naturalize and justify economic arrangements that are rooted in inequality? How does transnational surrogacy function as a site of racialization, and how do discourses of race and racial hierarchy unfold in transnational surrogacy? In the context of acute global and local inequalities, how is racial perception both built and accepted through assisted reproduction? To what extent does the racialized structure of transnational surrogacy become a means of justifying the unequal economic arrangements on which it is based?

And so I embarked on a journey to grasp how perceptions of racialized bodies inform surrogacy practices in India as well as ideas about kinship and relatedness. While the literature on transnational surrogacy at the time emphasized the centrality of local and global inequalities, including class, gender, race, and nation, these concerns were rarely the focus of analysis. This book pays special attention to the racial dimensions within transnational surrogacy, investigating how transnational surrogacy in India elicits new ways of thinking about race and racial formation, even in the absence of explicit discussions about race. These ideas inform surrogacy practices and have powerful consequences for how actors conceive of their relationships with one another. Yet while these constructions of race reflect stratified reproduction, they simultaneously complicate the concept, illustrating how actors may simultaneously challenge and reinforce structures of inequality. I theorize the ways in which transnational surrogacy relies on what I call *racial reproductive imaginaries* that reflect the values and meanings attached to ideas of race through which people imagine transnational reproduction. By exploring the ways in which social relations take on variable meanings by different actors, I contrast the various imaginaries enacted by commissioning parents, doctors, and surrogates. In doing so, I show that reproductive actors employ shifting and sometimes contradictory constructions of race to make sense of the transnational exchanges underlying family formation in the context of transnational surrogacy. Indeed, it is through such processes of racialization that actors imagine and embody kinship and family.

Transnational Reproduction and Surrogacy in India

In this book I use the term transnational reproduction to refer specifically to the transnational consumption of assisted reproductive technologies (ARTs). Also known as "reproductive tourism," "procreative tourism," or "fertility tourism," transnational reproduction centers on individuals who seek and provide a range of reproductive products and services. It includes people who travel abroad to procure gametes (sperm and eggs) and embryos, to contract with surrogates, and/or to obtain services such as IVF, intracytoplasmic sperm injection (ICSI), artificial insemination, sex selection, and diagnostic tools including amniocentesis and preimplantation genetic diagnosis (PGD). The providers of these reproductive tissues and services—including egg providers and surrogate mothers—may also undertake travel in order to make their bodies "bioavailable," to use a term coined by anthropologist Lawrence Cohen (2005).

In recent years, scholars have objected to the term "reproductive tourism" since it suggests travel for leisure, thereby trivializing the serious nature of infertile couples' quests for conception. Several scholars have suggested "reproductive exile" as a more accurate term, highlighting the plight of couples who travel involuntarily due to constraints in their home country (Inhorn and Patrizio 2009; Matorras 2005), while others prefer the more neutral "cross border reproductive care" (Blyth, Thorn, and Wischmann 2011). Following Monica Casper, I have found that the term "transnational reproduction" provides a more productive framing, as it focuses attention on the bodies, practices, technologies, and forms of capital that cross national borders (Casper 2011). Foregrounding transnational aspects also calls attention to how reproduction is stratified. Transnational reproduction includes all forms of transnational interactions and consumption patterns involved in assisted reproduction, including the cross-border movement of bodily materials.

As reproductive technologies have been disseminated globally since the 1980s, governments around the world approach regulation in different ways. Some countries prohibit certain technologies or procedures, such as PGD and sex selection, which public sentiment may oppose as being too close to engineering a perfect child, or egg donation and surrogacy, which impose a heavy physical burden on the donor or surrogate. Others have limited access to reproductive technologies by marital status, age, sexual orientation, or infertility status, while other guidelines aim to regulate the anonymity or financial compensation granted to gamete donors. As U.S. sociologist Arlie Hochschild has written, commercial surrogacy reflects a "highly complex legal patchwork" (2009). At one end of the spectrum are countries such as the United States, which imposes no federal regulations regarding reproductive technologies and where only seventeen of fifty states have enacted laws permitting surrogacy (Lewin 2014). At the other end are countries such as Germany, whose parliament has authorized strict guidelines regarding access to and use of reproductive technologies.

Such variations in policy reveal how politics and social power relations permeate technology and science. Scholars of science and technology studies have argued that technoscience is neither inherently objective nor neutral; rather, the prevailing worldviews, desires, and fears of society imbue and reinforce it (Gould 1981; Harding 1991). Further, social studies of technoscience demonstrate that social inequalities are reproduced, reinforced, and perpetuated by unequal access to technologies.

The same holds true for reproductive science and technology. While assisted reproduction has brought some people increased freedom and opportunity, making parenthood possible for infertile couples, single men and women, and gay and lesbian couples through artificial insemination, surrogacy, or IVF (Layne 1999; Mamo 2007; Ragoné and Twine 2000; Agigian 2004), advances in reproductive technology too have promoted and maintained certain power relations, notions of gender, and particular constructions of the family. Some scholars, for example, argue that these technologies re-essentialize women by reinforcing patriarchal roles and objectifying women's reproductive potential (Rothman 1989). Others reveal how ARTs strengthen the traditional patriarchal family by enabling infertile heterosexual couples to reproduce while many clinics have barred single people, gay or lesbian couples, welfare recipients, and other women who do not conform to patriarchal ideals of motherhood from having access to ARTs (Roberts 1997). Indeed, as assisted reproduction both "reproduces and also challenges the norms it is ostensibly aligning with," it has become "curiouser and curiouser" despite its widespread normalization (Franklin 2013, 221).

Perhaps most controversial among the selection of reproductive technologies is commercial surrogacy. Teman (2010) offers an insightful analysis of why surrogacy remains the least acceptable ART practice in several countries. For many nations, surrogacy is considered a cultural anomaly, generating unease by calling into question dominant cultural assumptions about families and mothers, two fundamental concepts undergirding society. Surrogacy provokes cultural anxieties regarding family by uncovering how families—built through assisted reproduction in the marketplace—are social constructs rather than biological fact. Moreover, while surrogacy breaks apart the "perceived unity of motherhood" (Teman 2010, 7) by deconstructing motherhood into genetic, gestational, and social maternities (Cussins 1998), it also challenges the ideology of motherhood that in many cultures assumes a durable and natural mother-child bond (Markens 2007; Ragoné 1994; Teman 2010). At the same time, gestational surrogacy reinforces notions of biogenetic kinship; given that Euro-American notions of kinship are biogenetically based (Schneider 1980), surrogacy has enabled many infertile couples to "chase the blood tie" (Ragoné 1996) in pursuit of biogenetically related offspring.

In this context, scholars and filmmakers have explored how actors make sense of their participation in surrogacy arrangements and their relationships with one another. While surrogacy has prompted debates in feminist, ethical, and legal spheres for decades, in recent years anthropologists and sociologists have contributed much-needed ethnographic scholarship that illuminates the impact of surrogacy on notions of motherhood, kinship, and labor (Hochschild 2012; Markens 2007; Rudrappa 2012; Teman 2010; Pande 2014c; Vora 2015; Majumdar 2014; Rudrappa 2015). Helena Ragoné's study of surrogacy agencies in the United States and Elly Teman's work on surrogacy in Israel demonstrate how women involved in surrogacy rely on narratives of "gift-giving" to downplay the commercial nature of their relationship with one another (Ragoné 1994; Teman 2010). In India, two documentary films, *Made in India* and *Google Baby*, highlight the experiences of couples who journey to India to hire gestational surrogates (Frank 2009; Haimowitz and Sinha 2010), while another, *Can We See the Baby Bump, Please?* spotlights surrogate women's experiences and ethical challenges to commercial surrogacy (Sharma 2012). Others, meanwhile, have prompted interdisciplinary conversations in disciplines such as bioethics, law, and anthropology in order to deepen our engagement with questions around work, law, citizenship, and coercion (DasGupta and Dasgupta 2014a).

Amrita Pande and Kalindi Vora make a major contribution to theorizing transnational surrogacy in India. In her book, *Wombs in Labor*, Pande uses the frame of labor as her starting point, illustrating the ways in which commercial surrogacy is "a form of labor that traverses the socially constructed dichotomy between production and reproduction"; it is simultaneously "gendered, exceptionally corporeal, and highly stigmatized" (2014c, 6). Yet rather than rely on images of victimized Third World women, Pande conducts a systematic evaluation of the choices women make in order to participate in the global reproductive market, demonstrating how women both comply with and resist regimes of labor. Vora too places labor at the center of her analysis in order to develop notions of affective labor and biocapital; she uses these themes to explain how forms of labor (including surrogacy work and call center labor) mark new forms of "exploitation and accumulation within neoliberal globalization but also rearticulate a longer historical colonial division of labor" (2015, 21).

Studies of assisted reproduction in India shed light on evolving notions of caste, kinship, and gender, and scholars have examined the ways in which ARTs are received and negotiated in Indian infertility clinics (Bharadwaj 2002; 2003; 2006). This book goes further, examining the expansion of the Indian fertility industry in dynamic relation to networks of reproductive actors situated in a range of virtual and actual locations. I treat transnational reproduction as an emergent social formation and not as a portrait of "Indian surrogacy." That is, rather than taking Indian "surrogacy" or "assisted reproduction" as my object of analysis, I examine the social imaginaries of global reproductive actors as they emerge at particular geographic, historical, and technological junctures. While scholars have previously analyzed links between ethnic belonging, nation, and kinship, fewer have linked kinship to race (Wade 2007). I bring these intersections to the fore by uncovering the nuanced sets of relationships between clients and surrogates. By complicating the intersections between race and kinship, I illustrate the ways in which the process of kin making relies on ever more flexible ways of imagining race. The converse is also true: race-making processes depend on more destabilized categories of kin. In other words, kinship in the context of transnational reproduction provides a revealing frame of reference for understanding race (and vice versa), demonstrating precisely how these categories are constructed and made flexible in ways that reinforce social stratification.

While previous scholars have illuminated concepts of kinship and labor in the context of surrogacy and assisted reproduction in India, few have centered on the shifting racial formations that emerge, particularly in transnational settings. I place race and racialization processes at the center of analysis, building on the concept of stratified reproduction to examine the kinds of racial imaginaries people use when making sense of their relationships with one another. By highlighting the intersections of race and kinship in the context of transnational gestational surrogacy, I elucidate the complex and unexpected ways in which transnational surrogacy reinforces stratification.

Stratified Reproduction and Racial Reproductive Imaginaries

With ongoing advances in reproductive technology, feminist scholars have paid close attention to what Shellee Colen, in her 1986 study of West Indian childcare providers and their female employers in New York City, called stratified reproduction (Colen 1995). Stratified reproduction describes the ways in which political, economic, and social forces structure the conditions under which women carry out physical and social reproductive labor. This labor is differentiated unequally across hierarchies of class, race, ethnicity, gender, and place in a global economy. As part of a movement to shift childbearing (biological reproduction) and domestic labor (social reproduction) from the sphere of the "natural" to the center of social analysis, the concept of stratified reproduction continues the feminist project of interrogating gender relations and gender inequalities, particularly within the arena of social and biological reproduction (Rapp 2001). Stratified reproduction is central to this book as it provides a lens through which to examine how systems of inequality influence individuals' reproductive practices, their experiences with and access to ARTs, and the choices available to them.

Stratified reproduction provides a theoretical framework within which issues connected to reproduction and stratification can be queried. Reproductive practices like transnational reproduction define certain racial, ethnic, and class groups as, for instance, more or less "modern," "responsible," or "worthy" (Colen 1995; Kanaaneh 2002; Mullings 1995; Maternowska 2000). Researchers have used this concept to describe how reproduction is stratified, particularly by race, class, and sexuality, and the power relations and discourses of motherhood, family, and childbearing that create opportunities and allocate resources, enabling some women to reproduce and care for their children while inhibiting others from doing so (Kanaaneh 2000; Mullings 1995; Roberts 1997, 2002; McCormack 2005). Population policies (Kanaaneh 2000; Petchesky and Judd 1998; Greenhalgh 2008; Lopez 2008; Maternowska 2000), the criminalization of women who use drugs while pregnant (Roberts 1997), and dominant representations of poor women and women of color as bad mothers (Mullings 1997; Roberts 2002; Davis 2009) reflect the social implications of stratified reproduction. Since the mid-1990s, there has been an expansion of scholarship on stratification in the context of ARTs (Ragoné and Twine 2000; Franklin and Ragoné 1998; Pollock 2003; Roberts 2009). Such work, for example, examines media framings of and public discourses around women's use of ARTs (Davis 2009; Markens 2012); how sperm and egg donation industries perpetuate a form of gendered eugenics (Daniels and Heidt-Forsythe 2012); and how gametes and embryos are stratified-marketed according to gender, place of origin, and donor characteristics (Whittaker and Speier 2010).

Transnational surrogacy in India reflects many of these inequities; in India as elsewhere disparities in gender, race, class, and nation place some women's reproductive projects above others' (DasGupta and Dasgupta 2010; Gupta 2006, 2012; Pande 2011). Pande (2014c) argues that surrogacy in India is an explicit manifestation of "neo-eugenics," drawing attention to the contradictions that emerge when the Indian government promotes fertility treatments as part of the medical tourism industry while simultaneously supporting smaller families and permanent sterilization for poorer families. In other words, when women compare their previous pregnancies to their experiences as surrogate mothers, they highlight the paradox of an industry built on "pro-natalist technologies [in] an otherwise anti-natalist state" (Pande 2014c, 35). These narratives concurrently reflect a global trend of "stratified motherhood" (Pande

2014b). Similarly, France Widdance Twine has conceived of commercial surrogacy as a form of "stratified contract labor" in which the women who "sell their uterus" to wealthier women and men "lack the economic, social, and cultural resources of the couple whom they serve" (2011, 16).

Moreover, Marcia Inhorn's work on reproductive tourism in the Middle East illuminates the global economy that empowers the spread of ARTs. Building on Arjun Appadurai's (1996) theory of global "scapes," Inhorn develops the concept of "reproscape," which involves "a distinct geography traversed by global flows of reproductive actors, technologies, body parts, money, and reproductive imaginaries" (Inhorn 2011, 90). New forms of gendered reproductive labor circulate within these reproscapes, as most reproductive "assistants" are women who bear the risks of hormonal stimulation, egg harvesting, pregnancy, and childbirth. Certainly, the "stratified reproscape" in which Indian surrogacy occurs is highly uneven, offering a powerful exemplar of how "some individuals, some communities, and some nations have achieved greater access to the fruits of reproductive globalization than others" (Inhorn 2015, 24).

Yet while much scholarship has acknowledged the ways in which race, class, and gender inequalities are embedded in transnational surrogacy, few have examined precisely how such concepts are constructed.[4] In her work on Indian call centers and surrogacy clinics, Vora emphasizes that racialization is a critical process to track "even in the contemporary moment in India's transnational labor history, which was primarily instantiated through British colonial practices" (2015, 11). But precisely *how* do various actors articulate and comprehend ideas about race? This book addresses this question by placing race and racialized bodies at the center of analysis, in order to evaluate the diverse ways in which actors construct and engage shifting notions of race.

In the context of surrogacy, concerns about race and heritability are coded in conversations about likeness and difference and often take the form of "resemblance talk" (Becker, Butler, and Nachtigall 2005). As Helena Ragoné found in her study of gestational surrogacy in the United States, surrogates and couples draw on beliefs concerning racial difference to resolve conflicting feelings about the child (Ragoné 1998). For instance, when Ragoné questions Linda, a thirty-year-old Mexican American pregnant with a child for a couple from Japan, about racial difference, Linda replies, "No, I haven't thought about the child as mine because she's not mine, she never has been. For one thing, she is totally Japanese" (1998, 125). Linda's remarks illustrate how ideas about race elicit questions about relatedness even when there is no genetic tie. Given the ways in which the relationship between kinship and blood is constantly reconfigured (Schneider 1980; Carsten 2004; Johnson et al. 2013) and persistent conceptions of race as something that is heritable and embedded in biogenetic substance, the intersections between race and kinship become especially salient in the context of transnational, transracial surrogacy, where people make explicit decisions about the "kinds" of children they want to have.

Indeed, race is a powerful organizing principle within transnational gestational surrogacy, and it is implied in its racial geography. Commissioning clients are primarily white and hail from countries in the global north. They travel across racial-ethnic lines in order to hire Indian surrogates and egg providers who primarily come from lower-caste, lower-class backgrounds. To be sure, not all ART consumers are white, and some are privileged people of color (e.g., nonresident Indians), while not all surrogates are lower-caste or lower-class. But even when intended parents and surrogates may share similar nationality or cultural background, this book addresses the ways in which ART providers and consumers carefully police other problematic borders, such as caste or religion.

Within this racial geography, I approach race as an "unstable and 'de-centered' complex of social meanings constantly being transformed by political struggle" (Omi and Winant 2015, 110). Sociologist Moon-Kie Jung (2006) draws on the works of both Omi and Winant and Benedict Anderson to envision race as a form of "imagined political community," one that represents an identity of interests; a way of seeing the world and identifying interests in which actors construct their identities in relation to race, class, or nation. Because transnational surrogacy relies on ever-changing racial identities and constructions, of particular interest are the ways in which various social groups become racialized in particular historical and social contexts. In the case of transnational surrogacy, an always-shifting intersection of identities (including religion, race, class, gender, and nation) functions as markers for the construction of racialized identities of imagined communities (see Baber 2004). Indeed I do not view race in isolation from other factors such as class, nation, or gender; however my primary concern is to think about how race intersects with other aspects of identity.

Thus, taking inspiration from Khiara Bridges's (2011) study of pregnancy in a New York City public hospital, this book locates transnational surrogacy as a site of racialization. Miles (1989) argues that racialization refers to the systematic ways in which meaning is attached to a number of factors (including phenotypic features) that serve to create social boundaries among humans. Similarly, Omi and Winant (2015) refer to "racial formation" as the "sociohistorical process by means of which racial identities are created, lived out, transformed, and destroyed" (109). The exact dynamics of this process varies; the social forces of racialization can be seen as the continual construction of different racialized groups which are constantly reworked and recategorized (Banton 1977; Miles 1989; Gould 1981).

In transnational contexts, these reimaginings of race and racial groups are linked to the differential distribution and struggles over power and wealth. Indeed, as Winant argues,

> Globalization is a re-racialization of the world. What have come to be called "North-South" issues are also deeply racial issues. The disparities in status and "life chances" between the world's rich and poor regions, between the (largely white and wealthy) global North and the (largely dark-skinned and poor) global South have always possessed a racial character. They are the legacy of a half millennium of imperialism. (Winant 2004, 131)

Thus, if globalization is a "racialized social structure" (Winant 2004, 131), it is within this structure that commissioning parents confront the transnational inequalities that privilege their capacities to become parents while relying on the reproductive labor of women in the global South.

This racialized social structure provides the setting in which reproductive actors rely on what I call *racial reproductive imaginaries* to make sense of their own and others' bodies as they engage in transnational surrogacy. Louis Althusser borrowed the Lacanian term "imaginary" for his theory of ideology, which he defined as "the imaginary relationship of individuals to their real conditions of existence" (1971, 162). In other words, the imaginary is the representation of reality that obscures life's material and historical circumstances. Marcia Inhorn (2011) has argued that "reproductive imaginaries" are among the flows of reproductive actors and technologies that traverse the global reproscape. For instance, imaginaries that highlight the "birth of 'miracle' babies" (Inhorn 2011, 90) foreground the procreative promise of IVF while masking the role that economic resources and cultural power play in structuring people's experience with and access to technology.

Taking this concept a step further, in this book I describe how the racial reproductive imaginary enables actors to envisage their reproductive endeavors in ways that conceal the operation of race. These imaginaries explain how actors signify and give meaning to their actions; key to these imaginaries are particular notions of race and difference that simultaneously influence notions of kinship and relatedness and mask the role that race plays in structuring unequal reproductive relations between commissioning parents and surrogates. While anthropologist Sallie Han (2013) has demonstrated how practices of literacy and consumption illuminate the ways in which families become imagined and embodied in U.S. women's experiences of "ordinary pregnancy," I show how practices of racialization shape kinship and family making. In other words, it is through processes of race making that surrogates, parents, and others imagine kinship and family. I argue that these processes of racial and kinship formation are central to actors' efforts to comprehend and justify their engagement in commercial surrogacy. In doing so, I uncover the specific racial reproductive imaginaries that underpin the unequal relations at the heart of transnational surrogacy. This book illustrates how actors constitute racial reproductive imaginaries through various transnational reproductive practices: through practices that "Other," through articulation of difference, and through the production and reproduction of power and stratification.

A Note on Nomenclature

The terminology used to refer to the participants in transnational reproduction is diverse, contested, and often reflects a particular stance on assisted reproduction. The terms are value-laden and vary in accordance with one's social position, culture, and discipline (Beeson, Darnovsky, and Lippman 2015). Many of them indicate a bias either in favor of or opposed to commercial surrogacy; indeed, as Pande (2014a) writes, they are "discursive tools" that selectively emphasize or deemphasize certain relationships or issues. Use of certain terms may reinforce or resist oppression, and Bailey (2011) calls attention to the dangers of "discursive colonialism" or the application to non-Western contexts of terms and frameworks that originate in the West.

Given that terminology around third-party reproduction is so disputed, the choice of terms I use in this book was not simple. Many scholars and activists prefer the terms "birth mother" and "gestational mother" to refer to the women who gestate and hand over the child at birth, calling attention to the maternal relevance of the woman's role. Others prefer the term "gestational carrier" to refer exclusively to the woman's capacity as someone who gestates a fetus for another, thus deemphasizing her maternity. In the Indian clinics and among the women I interviewed who worked as surrogates, everyone used the term "surrogate" to refer to the women who were contracted to carry pregnancies to term, while commissioning parents used the terms "surrogate" and "surrogate mother" interchangeably, as I do in this book.

The individuals who commission surrogate pregnancies are also referred to by several terms, including intended parents, intending parents, prospective parents, commissioning parents, and contracting parents. Some object to the term "commissioning parent" because of its emphasis on economic arrangements, preferring instead "intended parent" to emphasize the ways in which family making through assisted reproduction involves many intentional acts. In Indian clinics and policy documents, the term commissioning parent is primarily used, while the people who travel abroad seeking surrogacy services typically refer to themselves as intended parents. Thus, I use both commissioning parent and intended parent in this book.

In the context of egg donation, everyone I encountered referred to the women who undergo hormone stimulation and egg harvesting for payment as egg or oocyte "donors." Yet, to call these women donors would be a serious misnomer; their explicit task in this global reproductive economy is to sell their ova for a specified sum of money. Indeed, all the egg providers I spoke with, both Indian and some South African, said they pursued egg donation because of financial need. Thus, while I use the term "egg donor" because it is most commonly used throughout the industry, I also refer to these women as egg "sellers" or "providers," in order to call attention to the participation of purchasers and providers of ova in a wider global economy (Nahman 2008). Doing so confronts the discomfort that egg donation evokes, particularly for those disturbed by the commercial aspects of assisted reproduction. Identifying those who receive eggs as "purchasers" and women who provide them as "sellers" also highlights the positionality of participants. The prospective parents who commission surrogacy arrangements and donor egg IVF typically come from wealthier countries than those from which egg providers and surrogates originate. These distinctions underlie the complex ways in which global ova donation and surrogacy reflect broader patterns of stratified reproduction.

Toward a Transnational Methodology

To understand the links between race and kinship in transnational reproduction, I conducted field research in India over fourteen months between 2008 and 2010, with the majority of the research completed during 2010. I also conducted follow-up interviews in India in 2014 and in the United States in 2011 and 2014. The bulk of my fieldwork was done in Mumbai, with additional research trips to Delhi and Anand, Gujarat. While I designed my research to enable long-term immersion in the cultural settings in which gestational surrogacy occurs, I also was concerned with the transnational processes that drive the surrogacy industry in Mumbai. Thus, the prospect of how to define a given "field," access research participants, or limit my scope of inquiry remained daunting.

Within anthropology, there is a marked shift toward multisited research and away from narrow "area studies" approaches (Marcus 1995), and this book represents, quite literally, a border-crossing topic that requires mobility as well as online and "deterritorialized" research (Gupta and Ferguson 1992). As others have argued, the "field" as a discrete, bounded, and geographically specific site is a problematic construction in anthropology, and as anthropologists shift their focus to the processes of globalization and transnationalism, they too must confront the challenge of defining the scope and sites of inquiry (Gupta and Ferguson 1997). Thus, this book illustrates a shift from a focus on single nationalities and locations, going beyond binary constructions of sending and receiving locations, to examine multiple hierarchies of sites and subjectivities.

This chapter opened with the stories of Nishi and Eben because they not only reveal the remarkable contours of transnational reproduction, but also the various spaces in which it occurs. Eben, cosmopolitan and financially secure, stayed in upscale hotels when traveling to Mumbai. Nishi, on the other hand, lived in a simple one-room dwelling in a working-class area on the outskirts of the city. I regularly traveled between such spaces throughout my fieldwork. Consequently, my methodological approach was organized around the attempt to trace "networks" of actors involved in transnational reproduction in Mumbai. The actors in my study include doctors, commissioning parents, surrogates, egg donors, and medical tourism brokers, among others. The spaces through which these actors moved included fertility clinics, private hospitals, commissioning parents' accommodations in India (often in high-end hotels or full-service apartments), and surrogates' homes (typically in working-class areas of the city).

I faced the significant challenge of figuring out how to enter such networks, particularly in a city with a population of over 18 million inhabitants. I turned to the same solution that many commissioning parents and doctors rely on to establish initial connections with each other: the Internet. I drew on a variety of online sources in order to make initial contacts in the field, including doctors' websites, online surrogacy forums, and public blogs chronicling intended parents' surrogacy experiences. After initiating contact via e-mail with an intended parent or medical tourism agent, for example, we would often set up a video interview via Skype, where we would "meet" for the first time. In many cases, these initial Skype interviews were followed by face-to-face meetings in Mumbai or Delhi, or, in some cases, at the family's home in the northeastern United States, as several participants lived in the region where I was based post-fieldwork. Thus, it is worth highlighting how online spaces themselves became a primary "location" in which I conducted research, and how online relationships often set the stage for subsequent in-person meetings in India or the United States (and vice versa).

I also used the Internet to identify and contact doctors who practiced surrogacy in Mumbai, Delhi, and Anand. For these doctors, the

Internet and word-of-mouth recommendations were the main strategies by which commissioning parents would learn of their businesses; therefore many of these doctors had developed websites advertising their surrogacy plans to international clients. I made initial contact with doctors via e-mail or phone, and set up meetings with doctors during my first field trip in 2008. Interviews with doctors primarily focused on the structure of their surrogacy practices, the clients and surrogates they encounter in their work, the challenges and rewards of practicing surrogacy, and their thoughts on the ongoing policy debates around the regulation of ARTs. When I returned to Mumbai in 2010, I followed up with most of these doctors to understand how their surrogacy practices might have changed in the two years since my previous visit. During my main period of fieldwork in 2010, I focused my research on four clinics in which doctors allowed me to meet surrogates and intended parents. I should note that the clinics included in this study are self-selected by doctors who welcomed the presence of a researcher.

As Inhorn (2004) has noted, fieldwork in infertility clinics depends heavily on the goodwill of their gatekeepers. Thus, I recruited surrogates, egg donors, and intended parents in several ways. With respect to commissioning couples, clinic staff initially approached clients to see if they wanted to participate in the study; staff would then make introductions between interested clients and myself. I conducted interviews with intended parents either at the clinic or another location convenient for the parents (often their hotel or a nearby restaurant), and in many instances I was able to meet with intended parents several times during the course of their trip. These trips would typically last one or two weeks if they were at the beginning of the surrogacy process (which would involve the coordination of sperm/egg collection and embryo transfer). If the child had recently been born and the parents awaited the travel documents necessary to leave the country with their child, their stay in Mumbai might last longer, anywhere from several weeks to several months, depending on the parents' country of origin.

Since I interviewed parents at distinct moments and in various locations throughout their surrogacy process, I was able to capture how parents' perceptions and experiences of surrogacy shifted over time. My interviews with intended parents focused on topics related to personal and reproductive histories, decision making around aspects of surrogacy and/or egg donation, thoughts on their relationships with the various actors involved, and opinions on assisted reproduction in the context of racial, ethnic, national, and class differences. My goal in these interviews was to elucidate the social histories, biographies, and motivations of parents pursuing surrogacy in India, their ideas about biogenetic and social kinship, and their thoughts on the ethics and debates surrounding gestational surrogacy in India.

I also made initial contacts with many surrogates and egg donors through my relationships with doctors in the clinics. Clinic staff would first explain who I was and the topic of my research to women visiting their clinic; they would then introduce me to women who agreed to participate in the study. With the assistance of a translator, I conducted interviews in Hindi or Marathi, the languages most commonly used by the women. I found that, like intended parents, many of the surrogates or egg donors I met in the clinic were eager to meet again outside the clinic, and these meetings often led to introductions to other surrogates and egg donors.

Thus, I recruited a significant number of participants outside the clinic in women's homes, including surrogate agents. I use the term "agent" to describe women who recruit potential surrogates and egg donors for fertility doctors, and also care for surrogates during the duration of their pregnancies. While many of the women in this study are native speakers of Marathi and/or Hindi, they use the English term "agent" in conversation to describe this position. Similarly, agents used English terms such as "patient," "surrogate," or "donor" to refer to the women they cared for. One of my most enthusiastic interlocutors, Antara, herself a former surrogate turned agent, introduced me to many of her "patients" in her home over the course of my fieldwork. Often, as many as six or eight women would congregate in Antara's home during my visits, and our meetings frequently resembled a focus group, community-like atmosphere rather than individual interviews. These women would sometimes bring their sisters or children to the meetings; in a few cases, women brought their husbands. In other instances, I would travel with or without an agent to the home of a surrogate, where I would meet with the surrogate, her husband, children, and perhaps her parents or her husband's parents.[5]

Here, it is useful to note that there is very little privacy in Mumbai. My interviews with surrogate women and egg donors often included mothers, sisters, children, husbands, neighbors, and any other friends or family members who might be present in the home. Indeed, it would have been awkward to request privacy in the context of a one-room dwelling; there was simply no other place to go. Moreover, had I insisted on private interviews, it would have removed women from their cultural context to some degree, assuming the internal, individual self to be more genuine than their socially embedded self.

As Halliburton has shown in his study of mental illness in South India, such encounters reveal how a person is embedded in her social relationships; in contrast to the egocentric or individual self, in South Asia it is more accurate to speak of the socially dispersed or socially embedded self (Halliburton 2009). In my own work, women identified themselves in relation to others in their social networks: they were mothers, sisters, wives, and friends. Indeed, in interviews with families and groups of women, I noted that it was not just the women undergoing surrogacy but a "therapy managing group" of family, friends, agent, and fellow surrogates who are close to the patient (see Janzen 1978). However, while such interviews proved cathartic at times for women who opened up about family, marriage, and the challenges of surrogacy, I also noted several disadvantages to this method. Some women, for instance, would take my translator and me aside after an interview to express their "true" feelings about a surrogate, a family member, or their caretaker. Others might have felt hesitant about speaking critically about their family or their husband in front of others, particularly in a society where family unity is highly valued. I sought to mitigate these disadvantages by interviewing women multiple times over the course of my research, in order to build trust and to gather their opinions and experiences over time and in different settings.

By visiting women at their homes, I was able to observe how women interacted with each other and with their families away from the watchful eye of the doctor and clinic staff. This allowed me to grasp how surrogacy affected their everyday lives, in their homes, and with their families over the course of their pregnancies. My interviews with surrogate mothers focused on their personal biographies and motivations for becoming a surrogate or egg donor, their experiences with doctors and intended parents during the course of pregnancy, their thoughts on their relationship with the intended parents and the child conceived through surrogacy, and the ways in which surrogate pregnancy affected their everyday lives.

I supplemented the insights gained from interviews with participant observation throughout the encounters and spaces described above, which often included accompanying foreign visitors in their hectic travels across the city. For instance, I witnessed a "day in the life" of a traveling foreign egg donor, as she moved from hotel to clinic waiting room to the ultrasound room in which I observed the technician count how many eggs were developing in her ovaries. I also found that much of surrogate women's medical experience of surrogacy occurs outside the clinic, as I occasionally observed a caretaker administering hormone injections to a surrogate on the floor of her home. Field visits to surrogates' homes also offered opportunities to participate in activities not only as a researcher but also as a guest or visitor. Visits to Antara's home sometimes included an impromptu cooking lesson or an invitation to the wedding celebration of their landlord's daughter. These experiences generated much insight into the day-to-day lives of women in Nadipur.

My own positionality as an Asian American female anthropologist in the field affected my research in various ways. My Indian interlocutors often mistook me, a Filipina American, for a native of Nepal or the northeastern region of India. Thus, although I was a foreigner in India, many did not view me as "American," and this sometimes narrowed the perceived social distance between research participants and myself. Indeed, I believe this affected the willingness of some doctors to allow me to visit surrogate housing, which typically was located in areas where foreign researchers were uncommon and conspicuous.

Yet my U.S. nationality also positioned me as something of a curiosity for many participants, particularly the surrogates and their families, who, over time, felt comfortable posing questions about social life in the United States. Once my interlocutors accepted that I was indeed from the United States, the conversation often turned to all manner of questions about marriage, family, children, where my parents lived, how I met my husband, and whether he was from the same caste as I. In many cases women shared intimate details about their surrogacy experiences that would not have been considered proper to share in male company; thus, my position as a woman, with a female translator, was also advantageous. I also found that many intended parents visiting India welcomed the opportunity to speak with a fellow American or foreigner in the country. Many of these parents had no prior experience traveling in India, and they often appreciated the opportunity to speak with me and share experiences and thoughts about culture shock, life in India, and cross-cultural misunderstandings.

Lastly, I should indicate how my positionality as an anthropologist affected my reception in the field. During the years of my field research, there was a surge in media coverage of surrogacy in India. Thus, many doctors and commissioning parents were wary of speaking to a stranger about their surrogacy experience, as they did not wish to be profiled in any media outlets. I took great care to explain my position as an anthropologist (not a journalist) and I assured all participants that their comments would remain confidential. I also provided copies of consent forms bearing the institutional review board approval stamp for my research, as well as letters from my home institution in the United States and host institution in Mumbai. In many cases I found that these documents convinced participants, particularly doctors and parents, that I was not a journalist, and they subsequently felt more open to share "the whole story" of their experiences with surrogacy.

The Chapters to Come

The chapters in this book focus in turn on the various actors involved in transnational reproduction: the commissioning parents, doctors, and surrogate mothers who come together in the process of conceiving a child. Following a discussion of how transnational reproduction emerged in India in chapter 1 I focus on the narratives and experiences of intended parents in chapters 2, 3, and 4. Chapters 5, 6, and 7 emphasize the perspectives of doctors and surrogate mothers in India. Though the experiences of these actors clearly overlap, the individual stories of parents, doctors, and surrogates illustrate key points of each chapter and unveil the ways in which actors construct notions of race in transnational surrogacy.

Chapter 1 describes the emergence of India as a global surrogacy destination within a broader discussion of public health, assisted reproduction, and medical tourism. By critically examining the political-economic contexts of transnational reproduction, I consider the practice as a "racialized therapeutic landscape" that illuminates the sociopolitical dynamics within which gestational surrogacy has thrived. I suggest that in order to grasp the contemporary politics of reproduction in India, we must analyze the foundations of racialized politics of power in transcultural health care settings. I complement this analysis with a description of the range of clinics and surrogacy practices one may encounter in India. While I approach commercial surrogacy in India through a transnational lens, I also investigate the context of surrogacy "on the ground" in order to demonstrate how the construction of therapeutic landscapes produces and perpetuates certain stereotypes about race.

Chapter 2 examines how commissioning parents create and make sense of their relations with surrogates, egg donors, and the children born through surrogacy. How do intended parents narrate their family's origin stories? Within these narratives, what kinds of racial ideologies do they rely on? I argue that commissioning parents construct boundaries that position the surrogate as racially Other to themselves and their families, in ways that allow them to focus on Indian women alternately as objects of rescue or as shrewd actors involved in economic transactions. I suggest that these narratives serve to naturalize inequities between commissioning parents and surrogates in order to justify their participation in unequal economic arrangements.

Chapter 3 analyzes constructions of skin color and race in intended parents' narratives about the experience of selecting an egg donor. I show how egg donors of different backgrounds are differently valued, bolstering social hierarchies. At the same time, I describe the diversity of ways that intended parents approach race and skin tone when choosing an egg donor. I find that in contrast to dominant assumptions that intended parents seek donors who match their own ethnic backgrounds in order to reproduce whiteness, the process of egg donation represented an opportunity for many intended parents to subvert racial hierarchies by selecting Indian donors with darker skin tones. I argue that such narratives, however, misrecognize donor egg selection as an opening to challenge racial hierarchies; instead, such decisions rely on essentialized notions of race and beauty that exoticize Indian women and reflect new articulations of biological race.

In chapter 4 I examine the ways in which notions of citizenship and nationality intersect with ideas of race and kinship in the context of transnational surrogacy. With increasing numbers of people traveling from other countries to India in order to commission surrogate pregnancies, there have been reports of parents unable to obtain citizenship for their children born in India. This chapter explores what happens when incompatible national legal frameworks, policies about surrogacy, and practices of assigning citizenship intersect in the context of transnational surrogacy in India. I focus on the process of gaining citizenship in two countries that illustrate the range of approaches to transmission of citizenship: the United States and Norway. In particular, I analyze how ideas about citizenship and motherhood intersect with racial ideologies (related to blood and genes) to take on new meanings through transnational surrogacy processes. I argue that while assisted reproduction may expand conventional understandings of kinship and family, it also renaturalizes state definitions of citizenship and motherhood.

Chapter 5 offers an in-depth analysis of the key role that doctors play in organizing and facilitating surrogates' relationships with commissioning parents. By examining how doctors influence the ways in which surrogates themselves understand and negotiate their relationships with commissioning clients, I argue that Indian doctors racialize surrogates in ways that justify their unequal position in surrogacy arrangements. The chapter first addresses the ways in which doctors articulate their own role in transnational surrogacy arrangements, demonstrating how they structure relationships and facilitate communication between clients and surrogates. I then examine surrogates' narratives regarding their relationships with intended parents, demonstrating how physicians' practices powerfully shape how surrogates view their own relationships with commissioning clients and fetuses. I elucidate how physician racism and a racialized labor market shape surrogates' views of commissioning parents as actors in an economic transaction, rather than as co-collaborators in the creation of babies. Yet while doctors develop racial reproductive imaginaries through which they justify their treatment of surrogates, surrogates simultaneously describe this treatment as problematic and disrespectful, and perceive their inability to communicate directly with clients as a mark of disrespect.

Extending the discussion of physician racism in chapter 5, chapter 6 explores the ways in which doctors provide medical technologies and treatments to surrogate mothers, arguing that doctors racialize women who become surrogate mothers in ways that construct the surrogate mother and her pregnancy as always and already high-risk. I contend that this construction contributes to the justification of excessive medicalization in surrogate pregnancies; I show how doctors rely on practices of social control and excessive medicalization to control women's pregnancies, which culminate in soaring rates of cesarean sections among surrogate mothers. This chapter illuminates how gestational surrogacy and cesarean delivery are inextricably intertwined; these interrelated processes stem from practices that racialize this group of women as inherently risky. The chapter concludes with an analysis of the ways in which surrogates understand and negotiate these practices of medicalization and social control, focusing on their views and experiences of cesarean section.

Chapter 7 outlines the complexities of agency, constraint, and inequality in the lives of women who become surrogates in India. Women's personal narratives reveal the global surrogacy industry's reinforcement of a broader stratification of reproduction. They also show women's resistance to victimhood. In the context of physician racism and structural inequalities discussed earlier in the book, I analyze how women challenge racialized constructions of Indian surrogates to create new opportunities for themselves and their families, albeit within larger structures of power. I also examine the roles of women, many of them former surrogates, who act as intermediary agents. I show how the creation of intermediary positions reinforces the increasingly refined hierarchies inherent in transnational surrogacy. By revealing the many ways in which women exert (limited) power, I highlight the social divisions inherent in transnational surrogacy.

In the Conclusion, I reflect on the various themes discussed in the preceding chapters, elucidating the ways in which transnational surrogacy can be considered a technology of race. By viewing surrogacy as a technology of race and analyzing the ways in which racial reproductive imaginaries work to naturalize and maintain structures of inequality, this book shows how understanding the ways in which inequality becomes taken for granted is key to dismantling those very processes and the structures of which they are a part.

1

Public Health and Assisted Reproduction in India

I first met Karishma in Dr. Singh's office, where she was pursuing a second attempt at becoming a gestational surrogate. She was friendly and inquisitive throughout our brief conversation, and at the end of our interview she invited me to visit her at her home in Kailash, about an hour and a half outside Mumbai. I eagerly accepted.

I would soon learn that in contrast to many of the homes I had visited (which often lacked running water and many material possessions), Karishma's appeared perched on the edge of the middle class, belying dominant media representations of impoverished Indian women desperate to rent their wombs as surrogates. Indeed, while making plans to visit Karishma and her family, Karishma's husband inadvertently texted a shopping list intended for the local provisions store instead of the directions we needed to travel to their home. The list included items such as brand-name household supplies and Bournvita (a chocolate malt drink mix); reflecting her surprise at the shopping list, my translator remarked, "These are items we would buy ourselves," indicating that the family was closer to middle-class status than working class. My translator's hunch was confirmed once we arrived at Karishma's home; unlike some of the women I had interviewed who lived in small, one-room shanties, Karishma and her family lived in a two-room flat with running water. Various food provisions lined the pantry shelves, as well as a few children's toys. In the background, Karishma's two daughters were watching cartoons on a large television set, and in the center of the room Karishma set a plate of biscuits on the coffee table. After offering us snacks and refreshments, she sat down to tell us her story.

Twenty-nine-year-old Karishma was married and had two daughters, aged seven and three. She and her husband, Rajan, had both completed high school. While Rajan worked in the hospitality industry after completing a diploma in hotel management, Karishma described herself as a "housewife," though she had also previously studied nursing and had worked as an auxiliary nurse midwife. Yet, after the birth of her children, she said, "I had to think about who would take care of them," and she decided to stop working in order to care for her children.

Though Rajan could sometimes earn a monthly salary of up to U.S.$650, the family's finances were unstable. Rajan was in the process of starting his own hospitality consulting business with several colleagues and did not have a steady income. Karishma wanted to help her husband support the family and suggested that she might earn money as an egg donor or surrogate, which she had learned about from Rajan's sister, herself a former surrogate. Explaining his reaction, Rajan says, "I was against it then, but there were some financial messes. Checks were bouncing, and we were in need, so she said she wanted to contribute and help." Karishma too initially was somewhat uncertain, saying, "I kept wondering how such things [conception through egg donation or surrogacy] could happen." But eventually, she realized, "By doing this, we are getting some financial help. And there is no other place where such immediate financial help is available."

While Rajan was out of town for work, Karishma decided she would sell her eggs in exchange for approximately U.S.$260. She returned to sell a second time at a different clinic, earning the same amount of money. When she wanted to sell her eggs a third time, however, her doctor, Dr. Singh, suggested that she become a surrogate. As Karishma explained, "The doctor said that donors were not needed; surrogates were needed. 'Don't do donation now,' she said." Talking it over with Rajan, they decided to move forward with surrogacy: "We thought that if we got good money, we could add to our earlier savings and buy a house."

In the end, Karishma attempted to become pregnant as a gestational surrogate twice; embryos made from the intended father's sperm and an anonymous donor's eggs were transferred to Karishma's uterus. In both attempts, the client was a Russian man named Seth, whom Karishma met once, briefly. The first attempt ended in miscarriage early in the pregnancy, and the second attempt did not result in pregnancy. She earned about U.S.$220 for undergoing embryo transfer at each attempt, and the family ended up with little savings. Rajan explained that both times the couple had to commute long distances and keep both children in day care during Karishma's hospital stay—fifteen days following each embryo transfer. The costs of travel and childcare consumed a substantial portion of her earnings.

Karishma also described the surrogacy process, which included multiple injections of hormonal treatments over a period of weeks, as physically painful. She explained:

> During the process, surrogate mothers alone face the problems. The injections, which you take for about 15–20 days[,] are very painful. We can't sit; we can't sleep on one side. There are a lot of cramps after the injections. . . . I took forty injections the first time, which went on for about two to three months. It failed. There was so much pain. The second time I took 15–20 injections and again there was so much pain.

Furthermore, she was disappointed and disillusioned with the treatment she received from Dr. Singh, who, as we will see, Karishma believed did not fully inform her of policy changes that would affect her payment. However, when asked if she would ever try becoming a surrogate again, she replied that she would consider surrogacy with a different doctor, telling me, "You go to other hospitals [for your research]. If you hear of a good offer, let me know."

***

As Karishma struggled to gain access to the global surrogacy market, another family in Australia grappled with infertility and dreams of parenthood. Jan Marks was thirty-seven years old when she first met her husband, Stephen, in 2005. Two years later, Jan and Stephen were married and in the midst of expanding their home from two to five bedrooms; already a stepmother to her husband's sons from a previous marriage, Jan treasured her family and was eager to fill their home with two more children of her own. Aware of the difficulties women of her "advanced age" face in getting pregnant, the Australian couple immediately began trying to have children. After several years of multiple miscarriages and attempts at IVF, Jan learned that she had a bicornuate uterus, commonly referred to as a "heart-shaped" uterus, and that it was very unlikely that she would ever be able to gestate and give birth to a child of her own. Moreover, she learned that if they decided to continue pursuing parenthood through surrogacy, they would have to do so with donor eggs, as her own eggs were no longer a viable option.

Jan was devastated by this news but undeterred in her desire to become a parent. She turned next to adoption, but quickly realized that domestic adoption was "completely out" for them; in their native Australia, she explained, "we don't have adoption agencies that are private—and nobody adopts." Given the low rate of domestic adoption, they considered international adoption, yet grew disheartened when they learned of the long waiting periods and additional barriers due to their age and marital histories:

> There are very few domestic adoptions, so we looked at intercountry adoption. And because we had both been married before, our choice was narrowed down to one country. We don't have a good intercountry adoption system here and there are so, so many people wanting to adopt overseas. In our state, there were fifty couples inquiring every six months. To even get to the first waiting list, it was going to take eighteen months to get to the first interview. If we were successful, if we were allowed to even get into the program, it would have been seven years. And because I was thirty-nine at that stage, they basically said to me, "No chance!"

At this point, they briefly considered fostering, but quickly decided that fostering was not a good "fit" for them:

> One of the questions we were asked was, "Are you entering into fostering with the hope of having a child come to live with you?" And I could honestly not answer "no" to that because my intentions were that I would hope that I would have the child because I wanted to be a mother. And then we found out that a child would be taken away from us eventually and we'd be told not to have any contact with that child who had been with us—and emotionally we couldn't do that.

In 2008, believing they had exhausted all their options for expanding their family, Jan and her husband began to consider surrogacy with egg donation. While altruistic surrogacy—in which a surrogate is paid only for expenses incurred—is legal in Australia, commercial surrogacy—in which surrogates receive financial compensation—is considered a criminal offense. Knowing that there are very few cases of altruistic surrogacy in Australia, Jan looked to the United States, as she had not yet learned about surrogacy in India. Jan and Stephen were not exceptionally wealthy, but both were educated professionals, and while the surrogacy fees in the United States were prohibitive for most parents in my study (often costing upward of U.S.$80–150,000), Jan and Stephen were financially stable and keen to begin the process. They sold everything except their house, paid off most of their mortgage, and were ready to proceed.

Then, as the economic crisis of 2008 erupted, they realized their costs had grown well beyond their surrogacy budget. With surrogacy in the United States now out of reach, Jan canceled their plans, continued to do more research, and discovered surrogacy in India. Though her initial reaction was of denial and disbelief—Jan's first thought was, "No way in the world are we going all the way there and plucking poor Indian women out of the slums for surrogacy!"—she discovered online support forums and blogs that shared successful stories of parents returning home from India with babies born through surrogacy. Eventually, Jan and her husband thought, "If these people can do it, so can we," and they booked their first trip to India in 2008. Over the next two years, Jan and Stephen would make three more trips to India in order to attend two different clinics in Mumbai and Delhi before finally welcoming their son, James Alok, into the world in 2010.

***

The two stories above are very different: one of a struggling middle-class Indian family that turned to surrogacy and egg donation as a temporary solution to ease financial hardship and the other of a well-off Australian couple pursuing parenthood through Indian surrogacy. On the one hand, Karishma and Rajan's story mirrored that of many families who felt ambivalent about surrogacy or egg donation but pursued it anyway because of financial need. Though both had concerns about the process and Karishma had strong complaints about the physical toll egg donation and surrogacy took on her body, Karishma remained interested in the prospect of becoming a surrogate in the hope that she would meet a new doctor who would pay more. What motivates so many women like Karishma to become egg donors and/or surrogates?

At the same time, Jan's story, like those of many parents I interviewed in the course of this research, illustrates the ways in which parents eventually reach the decision to pursue surrogacy in India. Indeed, couples did not reach these decisions easily, and many were initially quite resistant to the idea of surrogacy in India, as was Jan. For many parents, the decision to pursue surrogacy is a difficult one, often following long histories of infertility and financial loss, and elucidates the range of ethical, moral, financial, and physical challenges at stake. In Jan and Stephen's case, their surrogacy journey included several IVF attempts and miscarriages, explorations into international adoption and fostering, significant financial losses from failed surrogacy plans in the United States, and finally several surrogacy attempts in two different clinics and cities in India. While the parents' stories uncover a range of motivations and personal histories with infertility and reproductive disruptions, how did they all end up journeying to India to hire gestational surrogates?

As commissioning parents and surrogates narrate complicated reproductive and personal histories, this chapter asks how India in particular emerged as a surrogacy destination for foreign prospective parents seeking babies and Indian women seeking an income. What is the constellation of contexts that makes surrogacy in India possible for both infertile couples pursuing parenthood and women seeking to become surrogates or egg donors? When and why did India surface as a leader in reproductive tourism?

In this chapter I address these questions by tracing the history and context of global medical travel for assisted reproduction in India. Indeed, this chapter provides the historical context necessary to understand not just the current state of reproductive tourism in India, but how and why India emerged as a major destination for reproductive tourists. I treat three topics: changes in health care accessibility for Indians, the rise of reproductive tourism, and efforts to regulate assisted reproduction in India. I place in historical context the emergence of India as a global surrogacy destination within a broader discussion of public health, assisted reproduction, and medical tourism, showing how the shift in health care priorities from primary health care to high-tech solutions set the stage for the growth of reproductive tourism in India. I then analyze the political economy of medical and reproductive travel in India, examining ART laws and regulation in order to show how India emerged as a key "therapeutic landscape" (Buzinde and Yarnal 2012) for travelers seeking ARTs. By investigating the political-economic contexts of reproductive tourism, I consider the practice as a "racialized therapeutic landscape" that unveils the sociopolitical dynamics within which gestational surrogacy has flourished. I suggest that in order to understand the contemporary politics of reproduction in India, we must grapple with the structural relations of power that characterize transcultural sites of medical tourism. For example, exploring the encounters between elite consumers of ARTs and local providers of ART services reveals the foundations of a racialized politics of power in transcultural health care settings. A critical examination of the dynamics that give rise to and emerge from such settings offers invaluable insights into the negotiation of power.

My second goal in this chapter is to point to the practices and practicalities that are integral to the experience of reproductive tourism in India. As many intended parents explained to me, one of the most challenging aspects of surrogacy in India is the complex coordination of multiple reproductive actors, including doctors, surrogates, and egg donors. For intended parents, surrogates, and egg donors, the surrogacy journey includes numerous attempts, negative test results, and miscarriages. Commissioning parents also make multiple trips to India, though surrogate women too may travel long distances from their homes to reach clinics in the city or other cities in India. As intended parents, surrogates, and egg donors navigate the process of transnational baby making, what is the range of practices that Indian clinics make available to international consumers of assisted reproductive technology? How do these clinics approach their work with Indian women hoping to become surrogates? As surrogacy relationships are facilitated across transnational spaces through Skype, email, phone, and the Internet, what is the context of surrogacy "on the ground" in India?

Thus, this chapter also contextualizes the practice of surrogacy in India, describing the range of clinics and surrogacy practices that an intended parent or surrogate may encounter. While commercial gestational surrogacy has blossomed into a multimillion dollar industry in India,[1] the current absence of any laws regulating surrogacy has resulted in the proliferation of surrogacy clinics throughout the country, with no governmental oversight regarding surrogacy recruitment, medical care, treatment, and costs. While I argue that reproductive tourism takes place in a transnational context, my goal in this chapter is to investigate the context of reproductive tourism in India. In doing so, I demonstrate how the construction of therapeutic landscapes perpetuates certain stereotypes about race that simultaneously locate India as a reproductive tourism destination and reinforce global stratified reproduction. While many actors involved in reproductive tourism, including doctors, policy makers, and intended parents, claim that transnational surrogacy is about creating families for infertile couples and supporting poor Indian women to help their own families, I argue that it is simultaneously about positioning India as a modern, safe space for foreigners seeking advanced medical technologies in their journeys to parenthood. Ultimately, in scaling up India's participation in the global medical tourism industry, the patterns and practices of surrogacy reinforce the hierarchical relationships that draw medical tourists to India in the first place.

From Public Health to Privatized Health

Surrogacy and assisted reproductive technologies encompass a range of public health concerns, and scholars have called attention to the potentially adverse health outcomes for surrogates and infants born through surrogacy (Knoche 2014). Thus, in order to comprehend how medical travel for assisted reproductive technologies gained purchase in India's private medical market, I begin with the context of public health in India, particularly with an examination of the ways that public health approaches shifted over time from the period prior to and following independence to the current, neoliberal India. Understanding such histories of public health in India are central to examinations of ARTs and transnational surrogacy, as they shed light on the dynamics that produce India as a global medical tourism destination.

Public health policy during colonial rule largely reflected an interest in maintaining the health of the Indian Army, particularly from the mid-nineteenth century, following the rebellion of 1857. While the British government in India established medical services meant for British nationals, the armed forces, and a few privileged civil servants, the majority of the Indian population was denied access to Western medicine (Roy 1985). This interest gradually led to a broader interest in the health of the general population, and then only in response to urgent health crises caused by unrest and social disruption related to colonial conflict (Amrith 2009). Though provincial health departments were established in 1919, neither health planning nor medical education was related to the health needs of the people. However, while colonial health policy was limited and focused primarily on addressing epidemics, the most substantial improvements in public health occurred in early twentieth-century British India. The establishment of panchayats (local governments) led to improvements in sanitation and decreased rates of cholera (Tinker 1954). The provision of clean drinking water at major sites of pilgrimage further contributed to the decline in cholera (Arnold 1993).

Notwithstanding these improvements, public health remained a low priority for the colonial state, which justified its sparse spending on public health by citing India's "naturally" high death rate and threats of Malthusian catastrophe if too much was done to reduce mortality (Arnold 1993; Davis 2001). Yet while the colonial state was ambivalent with respect to questions of public health, Indian elites began to politicize health in order to hold the state accountable. By the 1920s India's modernizing nationalists were arguing that only a representative national government could look after the health of the Indian people (Amrith 2009).

In the 1930s, then, while still under British rule, the National Planning Committee of the Indian National Congress prioritized the health of the population as part of a broader agenda of transformation from above. Subsequent initiatives, organized by the Health Survey and Development Committee in 1946, the National Health Survey and Planning Committee, and the Five Year Plans, highlighted concrete principles for public health in resource-limited settings. These principles emphasized comprehensive, holistic approaches to public health. They maintained too that public health must address the problems of the entire population and that the state must focus on issues that caused maximum mortality and morbidity. Finally, these initiatives asserted that public health solutions must account for the availability and costs of technology, and prioritized building and maintaining infrastructure for providing services (Banerji 2001). Throughout these initiatives, public health officials considered poor socioeconomic conditions (lack of sanitation, clean drinking water, nutrition, and housing) a major factor in health and well-being. Health planners, then, focused on addressing these conditions through development programs and primary health centers, which were intended to cover medical care, control of communicable diseases, maternal and child health, nutrition, health education, school health, environmental sanitation, and the collection of vital statistics (Roy 1985).

Within the Union Ministry of Health and Family Welfare, two technical departments—the Health Department and the Family Welfare Department—were charged with addressing health issues through a holistic approach. Welfare services—land and public housing, water supply, nutrition, and education, among others—were to be addressed together with health issues in order to manage health through overall development (Banerji 2001); this holistic approach gained traction in the two decades following India's independence from British rule in 1947. Yet despite an initial emphasis on comprehensive health planning, the health system slowly began to focus on the provision of medical care for specific problems, while welfare sectors were dealt with separately. Scholars have attributed this shift away from holistic approaches to several factors, namely, second-generation public health planners' emphasis on high-tech solutions, their dismissal of the intersections between living conditions and health, the socioeconomic conditions that fostered rural/urban disparities in health care, the prioritizing of services that cater to the elite, and the overemphasis on training medical doctors rather than paramedical and nursing staff (Qadeer 2002). As a result, the health care system shifted away from free primary health care toward concentrating on population control and technocentric solutions. This preoccupation with family planning led to a deep neglect of health services, which had been painstakingly built up over the first two decades following independence (Banerji 2004).

In 1978 the Indian government signed the World Health Organization's (WHO) Alma Ata declaration that defined comprehensive primary health care as the basic health service that is the core of affordable and need-based development. Yet despite this declaration to entrust "people's health in people's hands," in 1979 the political leadership in rich countries persuaded the leaders of poor countries to embrace an alternative approach to comprehensive primary health care: selective primary health care, which is the antithesis of primary health care. These "vertical" programs, limited to dealing with a few diseases at a time and purported to be cost-effective, were prefabricated, technocentric programs that caused further damage to an already battered health system (Banerji 2004). Later, the Structural Adjustment Programs (SAPs) of the 1980s and health sector reforms of the 1990s further reduced primary level care to grassroots services (Qadeer 2002). This shift illuminates the ways in which global economies influenced health planning in India. As neoliberal policies gained purchase around the world, the Indian government abandoned its own efforts to build a welfare state and accepted structural adjustment policies and health sector reforms that enabled international capital to penetrate its markets and secure new areas of investment, including health care provision and delivery.

These reforms engendered a key shift in public health approaches. While previous conceptions of public health were based on epidemiological needs and the principle of self-sufficiency, new approaches to public health relied on global finance to modernize and refashion health systems. Trade agreements such as the General Agreement on Trade in Services (GATS) and the Agreement on Trade Related Intellectual Property Rights (TRIPS) led to the liberalization of medical markets, privatization of public sector services, and promotion of technology transfer (Shaffer and Brenner 2004). At the same time, the promotion of medical tourism increased along with the number of medical students abroad, reflecting the attraction of the expanding medical markets for middle-class professionals. Meanwhile, doctors moved from the public to private sector, seeking higher pay, minimal state interference, control over working conditions, and higher status. Even when in state employment, many doctors continued to maintain private practices (Baru 1998; Venkataratnam 1973, 1987).

Currently the Indian health system relies on a mix of primary health village centers and government hospitals to provide free medical care for the general population. Primary health care clinics offer services including immunization, treatment of common illnesses, prevention of malnutrition, and pregnancy, childbirth, and postnatal care. Patients needing specialized care are referred to secondary and tertiary care centers (Worthington and Gogne 2011).

However, while the public system seeks to make health care accessible to all, this does not always happen in practice. Parallel to the public sector is a private medical sector that caters primarily to the urban population and those in higher socioeconomic groups. Yet both urban and rural households tend to use the private medical sector rather than the public, with nearly two-thirds of all households seeking health care from the private medical sector. The most common reasons for not using public sector health care facilities are poor quality of service and unavailability of a facility nearby. Despite the rise of a number of insurance programs, only 5 percent of households report being covered by any kind of health insurance (IIPS 2007).

The poor feel the consequences of this decay in government health services most acutely. With fewer government services and with poor coverage, about 70 percent of Indians pay for healthcare and medications out of pocket, in comparison to 30 to 40 percent in other Asian countries such as Sri Lanka (WHO 2012; Sinha 2011). Catastrophic medical expenses can force patients and their families to go into debt, sell their assets, or halt essential medical treatment. Such health care costs lead to the increased vulnerability of the poor and a vicious cycle between good health and malnutrition, as families must choose between food and health care (Duggal and Amin 1989).

The effects are also seen in the quality of and access to maternal health care. In the 2005–06 National Family Health Survey, many women reported not receiving any high quality maternal health care; of mothers who had a live birth in the five years preceding the survey, only 44 percent reported starting prenatal care in the first trimester of pregnancy. Just over half of mothers (52 percent) had three or more prenatal visits. Ultrasounds were used in one-fourth of all pregnancies, while only 39 percent of births took place in health facilities.[2] More than half took place at women's homes, and about six in ten women did not receive any postnatal care (IIPS 2007). Women in this study who serve as surrogates, however, receive high-quality and highly medicalized treatment in their surrogate pregnancies, when they bear children for other parents-to-be.

In the new market framework, multinational corporations determine health priorities by controlling the availability of technologies. While this framework puts the individual needs of a small paying minority first, the state's responsibility for public health recedes in the public/private mix, justified in the name of "plurality of services" and "decentralization." The complex integrated health system has fragmented, forcing service institutions to rely on the operational principles of institutional economics and to abandon the holistic, systemic perspective. As health services became increasingly commodified and unequal, institutions invested in services that enhanced profits (such as orthopedic, cardiovascular, and obstetric services). Consequently, the poor encountered increasingly difficult access to quality health services. This system set the stage for the expansion of assisted reproduction and the medical tourism industry in India.

A Short History of Assisted Reproduction in India

On July 25, 1978, the world's first "test-tube" baby, Louise Brown, was born in the United Kingdom through the efforts of Dr. Robert G. Edwards and Dr. Patrick Steptoe. Brown was conceived through in vitro fertilization (IVF), an assisted reproductive technique requiring trained medical personnel and specialized facilities. To reproduce through IVF, women first take hormonal drugs that induce the production of multiple ova (rather than the single ovum that is produced in each cycle); a trained physician extracts these ova through a surgical procedure. The ova are then fertilized with sperm "in vitro" (in a laboratory) and allowed to grow into the embryo stage, when these embryos are transferred back into the woman's body. Often, women may take additional medications to increase the chances of embryo implantation. Dr. Edwards won the Nobel Prize in Physiology or Medicine in 2010 for his role in pioneering this assisted reproductive technology.

Louise Brown and Dr. Edwards are famous; few Westerners realize that only sixty-seven days after Brown's birth, the world's second and India's first IVF baby, Kanupriya Agarwal, was born on October 3, 1978 in Kolkata (then Calcutta). A team headed by Dr. Subhas Mukherjee conceived in vitro and delivered Kanupriya, referring to her with the pseudonym "Durga," after a Hindu goddess who embodies the female creative force. Initially the news was received with great interest and Mukherjee discussed the achievement in the press and on television, as well as at the Indian Science Congress. But the Indian government was skeptical and convened an official scientific committee—one that included no specialists in reproductive science—charged with evaluating Mukherjee's work. He was barred from presenting his work to the international scientific community, humiliated, and professionally harassed. He committed suicide in 1981 (Anand Kumar 2003).

By 1984 the scientific community had changed its assessment of IVF. The Indian government established an IVF program in collaboration with the King Edward Memorial Hospital, a tertiary care center of the Bombay Municipal Corporation at the National Institute for Research in Reproduction (NIRR), an institution of the Indian Council of Medical Research (ICMR). Doctors tested the technology on poor women seeking infertility services in this government hospital, and the first documented "test-tube" baby in India was born to the wife of a municipal employee on August 6, 1986. Seventeen years later, and twenty-five years after the birth of Durga, the Indian scientific community finally recognized Dr. Mukherjee's achievement (Anand Kumar 2003).

It may seem odd that the development and promotion of contraceptive technologies occurred jointly with the technologies of assisted conception in India. The nation's population control agenda has been one of the most central factors influencing women's experiences of childbirth and reproductive health in India since the early twentieth century. Historically and globally, apart from condoms and vasectomies, modern contraceptive technologies (e.g., the pill, the diaphragm, intrauterine devices, tubal ligations, Depo Provera, and Norplant) have been designed primarily for women's bodies. In India the development and distribution of contraceptives is not only gendered, but also classed. From its inception, the contraceptive pill received little attention in India, as it was viewed as suitable only for women in the global North and for upper class, educated Indian women. The lower class female was assumed to be incapable of controlling her own fertility (Jolly and Ram 2001). As a result, tubal ligation remains the foundation of family planning in India. In the 2005–06 National Family Health Survey (NFHS), female sterilization was cited as the most widely known method of contraception among women (97 percent), while only 61 percent of women reported knowledge of the IUD, pill, and condom (IIPS 2007, 113).

Thus, the expansion of ARTs in the context of aggressive population control programs illustrates a paradox: while government expenditure on public health infrastructure shrinks and population control programs target poor women, Indian scientists invest their efforts in the profitable and growing ART industry. Moreover, both technologies represent ways to control women's reproduction, either to prevent them from having a child or to exert social pressure on them to procreate. Indian reproductive experts Chander Puri, Indira Hinduja, and Kusum Zaveri, all of whom have been affiliated with NIRR, offer a curious justification for spending public money on this experimental procedure: for women who had undergone tubal sterilization, a widely used method for fertility control, IVF is a simpler, less invasive method of conceiving than tubal recanalization (Puri, Hinduja, and Zaveri 2000). In doing so, the authors claim they made sterilization more palatable for many Indians and that it is an enormous windfall for the Family Planning Programme. At the same time, the Declaration of the International Conference on Population and Development emphasized expanding the scope of reproductive health to include infertility, and thus promoted ARTs in the name of women's choices and rights.

This vision of ARTs—in which IVF represented a solution not only for infertile couples desiring children but also for couples seeking to reverse tubal ligation—joined promoters of the medical market interested in generating profits through ARTs to the pro–population control lobby of professionals and policy makers. At the same time, fierce infighting and ego clashes led to the demise of the NIRR's public sector IVF program. One researcher, for instance, spoke of the "arrogant" and "uncompromising" attitude of the doctors; ultimately, the project suffered from a toxic climate of frustration due to conflicts between self-interested "publicity-hungry individuals" and "disgruntled" researchers who felt their work went unappreciated (Bharadwaj 2002, 327). By the end of the 1980s, scientists involved with the program had left their government posts to set up private practice and the private sector almost completely took over ARTs. They became part of the glamour technologies India projected to establish its position as a leader in the international medical marketplace (Qadeer 2010). At the same time, media narratives that functioned as publicity-driven "institutional advertisements" created persuasive images of expertise and achievement in the community of IVF practitioners; these narratives played a critical role in the commercial success of assisted conception in India (Bharadwaj 2000).

As the use of IVF grew apace, surrogacy became a well-known option for infertile couples in the early part of the twenty-first century. The surrogacy boom started in 2004 in Anand, in the western state of Gujarat. A U.K.-based Indian couple, Aakash and Lata Nagla, had been suffering from infertility and Lata's parents approached Dr. Nayna Patel for help.

While Lata suffered a rare genetic condition that causes the uterus to develop abnormally, her eggs and ovaries functioned perfectly. Through IVF, Dr. Patel created embryos with Lata's eggs and Aakash's sperm, and then transferred the embryos into another woman's womb—that of Lata's forty-four-year-old mother. In 2004, Lata's mother gave birth to her own grandchildren, a twin boy and girl. Since then, the surrogacy industry has flourished.

Throughout the early decades of the twenty-first century, thousands of foreign couples traveled to India each year to take advantage of commercial gestational surrogacy.[3] The promise of ARTs often exploits intended parents' hope and optimism. Though many clients become aware of low success rates through painful experience (70 percent of clients will receive negative pregnancy test results) they tended to view Indian surrogacy as a smart, financial move in the gamble of IVF and surrogacy. Commissioning parents I interviewed calculated that if they could afford to spend U.S.$100,000 on surrogacy, their budget would go significantly further in India, where their funds would cover up to three surrogacy attempts, thus increasing their chances of bringing home a baby.

Today, India is a global hub of commercial gestational surrogacy. Infertility clinics can be found in urban megacities throughout the country; in addition, smaller towns and rural areas have infertility centers that work with ART centers located in cities where specialists perform IVF and ICSI (intra-cytoplasmic sperm injection) procedures. While international travelers visit surrogacy clinics in a wide range of cities, including Delhi, Mumbai, Hyderabad, and Anand, a growing number of IVF/surrogacy clinics in metropolitan cities throughout India cater to regional clientele from Bangladesh and Pakistan, as well as clients from within India, who travel from regions where ART infrastructure remains undeveloped (Kashyap 2011).

Creating Racialized Therapeutic Landscapes

Amidst the expansion of assisted reproduction, medical tourism—travel for medical care—has grown steadily in India and around the world. Patients have long traveled around the world seeking medical services; recent anthropological work suggests that the new transnational world order has increased medical migrations (Thompson 2011). Several recent special issues of anthropology journals have been dedicated to the theme of medical travel, highlighting empirical studies of transplant tourism, plastic and sexual reassignment surgery, stem cell tourism, and vacation travel to various healing spas (Mazzaschi and McDonald 2010; Naraindas and Bastos 2011; Roberts and Scheper-Hughes 2011; Whittaker, Manderson, and Cartwright 2010). While several countries throughout Latin America and Asia actively promote medical tourism, including Cuba, Jordan, Malaysia, Singapore, and Thailand, India is one of the world leaders in medical tourism, second only to Thailand (Pande 2011).

There are several factors that position India as a desirable destination for such travel: inexpensive costs, well-equipped private clinics, and large numbers of well-trained English-speaking doctors with training from prestigious schools in India and abroad. Moreover, a significant overseas population of nonresident Indians avail themselves of medical care in India, often seeking cheaper medical treatment when they return to India for family visits. Indeed, medical tourism receives full government support; in 2004, the government launched an international advertising campaign and declared that medical treatment of foreign patients is legally an export and eligible for all fiscal incentives extended to export earnings. Most medical travelers to India receive cardiac care, while an increasing number of patients receive joint replacement, plastic surgery, eye treatment, and dental work (Pande 2011).

Interestingly, however, while researchers, news media, and participants in my own study cite low cost as a key factor in international medical travel, the promotion and marketing of medical tourism rarely highlights this issue. In a study of promotional print materials distributed at the first medical tourism trade show in Canada in 2009, researchers found that when marketing India as a global destination for medical treatment, marketing materials downplayed the cost issue in favor of emphasizing safe and advanced treatment facilities, as well as quality of care (Crooks et al. 2011). Indeed, in order to overcome negative images of health care in developing nations, the Indian government has focused on messages related to accreditation, on-site technologies, overall quality, and patients consulting with highly trained doctors, effectively demonstrating that the quality of care is on par with that in developed nations. Such efforts extend beyond the marketing of health care to include the enhancement of travelers' experiences from the moment they arrive in the country. In 2003, for instance, when then-finance minister Jaswant Singh called for the country to become a "global health destination," he urged the government to improve airport infrastructures in order to ease the experience of medical tourists (Chinai and Goswami 2007).

However, in examining the construction of India as a global health destination, I turn to therapeutic landscapes as a conceptual framework through which to understand the link between place, history, and health. While landscape holds various meanings, I take landscape to be a "text to be read for what it says about human ideas and activities" (Gesler 1992, 736). In other words, a critical examination of the emergence of medical tourism in India must attend to the sociopolitical and historical dynamics that construct India as a therapeutic landscape, as well as the relations of power between sending and receiving, or core and periphery, nations. As Buzinde and Yarnal (2012) argue, destinations of medical tourism produce therapeutic landscapes that are informed by neoliberal ideologies. Such landscapes unavoidably depict contemporary power relations and issues of inequality. Given that many medical tourism destinations are located in postcolonial regions, scholars must incorporate a postcolonial perspective in order to understand how therapeutic landscapes are "intricately linked to the histories of exploitation that once characterized and still define present day global relations" (Buzinde and Yarnal 2012, 784).

Viewing transnational reproduction through this lens illuminates the ways in which medical tourism in India constructs *racialized therapeutic landscapes* that are deeply stratified along racial and other lines. Reproductive tourists from the global North appear to transgress racial borders when they hire an Indian surrogate to gestate a "white" fetus, calling attention to racial difference, the reification of biological race, and assertions of racial privilege. Understanding transnational surrogacy in India as a racialized therapeutic landscape elucidates the ways in which "landscapes of healing are differently (re)produced for various segments of the global population" (Buzinde and Yarnal 2012, 785). In other words, racialized therapeutic spaces shed light on how notions of race are normalized and reinforced, emphasizing the ways in which therapeutic landscapes perpetuate racial stereotypes between core and periphery nations.

Regulating Surrogacy in India

Within this context, transnational reproduction has mushroomed in India, making the country the "mother destination" (Rudrappa 2010). Indeed, India represents a particularly interesting site because it is the first developing country with a burgeoning industry in transnational commercial surrogacy, in part because of lower costs but also due to minimal legal or regulatory frameworks for the provision of assisted reproductive technologies (ARTs) such as in vitro fertilization, egg donation, and gestational surrogacy.[4] These variables—the absence of laws governing ARTs in India, the relatively low cost of services, and the transnational clientele— have influenced the expansion of ART services in India aimed specifically at global consumers, and the attendant implications for understanding race and kinship relations within global reproductive networks.

Throughout the first decade of the twenty-first century, the complete absence of regulations in India drew many clients. The first reference to ARTs in a government document appeared in the "Ethical Guidelines for Biomedical Research on Human Subjects" published by the ICMR in 2000. In 2002, the ICMR and the Ministry of Health and Family Welfare (MOHFW) developed guidelines on the Accreditation, Supervision & Regulation of ART Clinics in India, which were later published in 2005. These guidelines, however, are not legally binding and no governing body implements them. Clinics decide whether to accept or reject the recommendations made in the guidelines, and effectively operate in the absence of any form of regulation of ARTs.

With the growth of medical travel for ARTs and gestational surrogacy, doctors and other stakeholders have pressured the Indian government to pass a law regulating ART clinics. In 2008 the ICMR and MOHFW outlined the Draft Assisted Reproductive Technologies (Regulation) Bill and Rules, which attempted to address many of the issues related to the regulation of ART clinics, semen banks, and research on embryos. The Draft Bill, a 135-page document, lays out the obligations of ART clinics (including duties regarding gametes and embryos, preimplantation genetic diagnosis, and sex selection) as well as the rights and duties of patients, donors, and surrogates. However, the 2008 Draft Bill came under attack from various groups, as it seemed to promote the interests of the private sector providers of the technologies rather than regulate them, and included few clauses designed to protect and ensure the health and well-being of women and children (Sama 2010; Sarojini and Sharma 2009). For example, it states that "ARTs carry a small risk both to the mother and the offspring" (Ministry of Health and Family Welfare 2008, 67) although gestational surrogates face increased risk for multiple gestation, ectopic pregnancy, and preterm birth.

In 2010, the ICMR released a revised version of the Draft Bill, devoting a substantial section to the regulation of surrogacy arrangements. Yet, as the organization Sama (which means equality in Sanskrit) underscored, significant gaps remain with respect to the protection of surrogate women. Most striking are the changes in the provision for payment to the surrogate woman, which undermines her rights and favors the intended parents. In the 2010 Draft, payment to the surrogate is to be disbursed in five installments (instead of three, as in the 2008 Draft) and 75 percent of the payment is to be paid at the fifth installment, following delivery of the child (in contrast to the 2008 Draft, in which 75 percent was to be made at the first installment). This move not only clearly prioritizes the concerns of the intended parents and doctors, but downplays the risks associated with surrogate pregnancy, labor, and related emotional and physical risks. The Draft also increases the number of permitted live births for a surrogate from three to five, inclusive of her own children, belittling the real threat to surrogate women's health by repeated pregnancies (Sama 2011). Moreover, public debate surrounding the Draft selectively represents the interests of the medical community that drafted the bill, with little mention of the surrogates and the health risks they bear (Majumdar 2013).

Concern also extends to whether the 2010 Draft excludes single people and gay couples, a subset of prospective parents who have been welcomed in certain Indian clinics. Some have argued that the language in the Draft, which allows "unmarried couples" and "single persons" from India and abroad to have children through gestational surrogacy, opens the path for gay couples and single people (Prakash 2010). Yet others suggest that because the Indian state does not recognize gay relationships, gay couples from India or abroad will not be permitted to use ARTs or surrogacy (Wade and Walters 2010).

While debates continued around the language of the 2010 Draft Bill (which still awaits consideration in Parliament), in December 2012 the

Ministry of Home Affairs first step toward regulating the practice of surrogacy and restricting its use to married couples. The ministry, noticing that many foreigners were entering India for surrogacy on tourist visas, stated that such foreigners should only enter India on medical visas. Moreover, such "surrogacy visas" would only be issued if the couple met certain conditions: first, they would need to supply a letter from their country's foreign ministry or embassy in India certifying that their country recognizes surrogacy, assuring that the child or children born to the Indian surrogate would be allowed to enter their country as the child of the couple. Second, only a heterosexual couple married for two years is eligible for the surrogacy visa (Rajadhyaksha 2013). The ministry came under attack by various groups for its apparent concern with gay couples' use of surrogacy while women's health risks remain unaddressed.

During my fieldwork in 2008 to 2010, many clinics saw a surge in the numbers of single people and gay couples seeking surrogacy; indeed, roughly half of the intended parents I interviewed were gay couples or single people. Yet amidst the government's concerns about surrogacy for gay couples and feminist concerns about the potential exploitation of surrogate women, many believed that transnational surrogacy in India was a profitable business and unlikely to end anytime soon. However, in late 2015 the government proposed a new law that would limit surrogacy services to Indian couples, effectively banning commercial surrogacy for foreigners (Shankar 2015). While the government claimed the ban was intended to combat the exploitation of poor women who work as surrogates, women's rights groups remain divided in their support of the ban, with some arguing it will make women more susceptible to ill-treatment (Malhotra and Sugden 2015). These guidelines and proposed legislation reflect the ever-changing landscape in which surrogacy arrangements take place.

Thus far I have focused on the history and political-economic context of assisted reproduction and reproductive tourism in India. Within this context, the lack of any legally binding regulations not only resulted in the proliferation of IVF clinics throughout India but, I argue, also set the stage for the expansion of practices that maintain structures of stratification. Below, I examine the structures and process of surrogacy as it unfolds across many stages, spaces, and with the participation of multiple actors.

Transnational Structures of Surrogacy

Prior to her first trip to India in late 2008, Jan Marks hoped to have a child that looked like her, so she made arrangements with a South African egg donor agency to send a young white egg donor to India. But just as the egg donor was about to travel to Mumbai with five other donors from South Africa, the Mumbai terror attacks occurred on November 26, 2008. Throughout the city, attackers carried out twelve coordinated shooting and bombing attacks, killing 164 and wounding at least 308 people. In the wake of these attacks, Jan learned that the South African agency had canceled the egg donors' trip, thus putting on hold the IVF cycle that was timed for Jan and her husband's visit. Faced with the decision of postponing their trip until their donor could reschedule her trip from South Africa, continuing with their December travels, or canceling their plans altogether, Jan and her husband decided to move forward with their plans:

> Everything was cancelled because it was too dangerous for the donors to go and we were absolutely devastated. But we had all our travel plans ready, so we decided we would go, ourselves. We would go and check it [the surrogacy clinic and process] out for ourselves, and if we didn't like what we saw then we would just quit it and that would be it. So we went to Mumbai and we had a great time. We realized that it was all above board, and we actually met the surrogate [who would carry the pregnancy] when we signed the contract, which was a really nice experience. We realized that no, she was not pulled out of the slums, that she was from the equivalent of a working class family. And so we signed our contracts and then our donor flew back [to Mumbai] in February as well. We didn't have to but we thought, This is just so weird and crazy, that we would at least like to be in the same country as our child when it is conceived. Not everyone's got the option to do that but we did because we sold everything and we had budgeted and we had a hell of a lot of frequent flyer points.

At this point, Jan's surrogacy journey, which had only just begun, displays the multiple levels of organization and communication required in order to arrange surrogacy in India. Jan's plan included the travel of an egg donor from South Africa; this meant that the doctors in India had to ensure that the cycles of the Indian surrogate mother and the South African egg donor were coordinated so that the egg retrieval, IVF, and embryo transfer could occur within days of each other. With the Mumbai terror attacks leading to the postponement of the egg donor's trip in November, Jan's hopes for a December pregnancy vanished. Yet while many parents might have considered abandoning the process altogether, Jan was determined to move forward with their surrogacy plans, despite the difficulties and delays she encountered and even in the wake of the devastating attacks in Mumbai.

Why did surrogacy in India remain Jan's preferred option, despite the many challenges she encountered? What are the surrogacy practices that draw parents to India, even in the context of national tragedy and turmoil? I return to Jan's story because, in order to comprehend why India exists as a global destination for transnational surrogacy, it is important grasp the current context of surrogacy in India, including clinic practices regarding surrogacy agreements and medical treatment that allow women like Jan to tailor surrogacy arrangements to their individual requirements. As mentioned earlier, low costs and lack of regulation, among other factors, made India an attractive destination for parents seeking gestational surrogacy arrangements. Yet economics and the absence of regulation were not the only forces compelling foreign clients to travel to India. In India, gestational surrogacy—in which the surrogate contributes only her womb, no genetic material—is the norm, and this allowed Jan to control the genetic makeup of the child. As a woman who would be unable to provide her own eggs, Jan did what she believed to be the next best thing; she worked with an agency in India that had connections with an egg donor agency in South Africa that would be able to provide white egg donors, at a fraction of the cost in the United States.

Paths to Surrogacy

What are the transnational structures of surrogacy that draw so many foreign couples to India? In this section, I describe the unique context of surrogacy in India, which in part allows clinics the freedom to determine their own practices in the absence of any laws or regulation. I suggest that this context attracted Jan and many parents like her to

India rather than other countries with burgeoning surrogacy industries, and that clinic practices rely on and reproduce social stratification at the local, national, and transnational levels.

While the clinics I visited had many differences in terms of their surrogacy practices and policies (which I will address in the last section of this chapter), the general stages of surrogacy are similar. For intended parents, the first step is to select an agency or clinic, as foreign couples almost never contract with an Indian surrogate mother independently. The doctors select the surrogate, not the parents. Virtually all parents rely on the Internet in order to make their decisions: they email prospective doctors and fellow parents who share their experiences of surrogacy in India, they join forums dedicated to surrogacy in India, and they read the many surrogacy blogs chronicling intended parents' surrogacy journeys to India. As they gather information on different clinics in different cities in India, among the strongest factors they take into account are the testimonials of other parents who have attended that clinic. Other key factors include cost, communication with doctors, and perceived treatment of surrogates. In general, commissioning parents in my study cited total surrogacy costs ranging from U.S.$20,000 to U.S.$40,000, which includes medical procedures, recruitment and care of the surrogate, surrogate housing, and hospital fees. Some parents saw their costs rise above this range when they were responsible for additional fees such as extended hospital care for complications resulting from premature birth, or longer stays in the country due to delays in acquiring travel documents after the birth of the child. Notwithstanding these additional fees, intended parents viewed surrogacy in India as a bargain when compared to costs in the United States, for example, where surrogacy costs range from U.S.$80–120,000, with some agencies charging upward of U.S.$150,000.

As clients progress through the initial phases of selecting an agency, agencies are constantly recruiting and screening potential surrogates. First and foremost, the pay draws women to surrogacy: most surrogates in this study reported receiving payments between U.S.$5,500 and U.S.$7,500, equivalent to several years' household income for most families. It is difficult to track the number of women involved in gestational surrogacy, and because a high percentage of surrogate births are multiple births, the number of live births is not a reliable predictor of the number of birthing women. Dr. Patel, of the Akanksha clinic in Anand, reports that at any given time 60 to 65 women contracted by her agency are pregnant, carrying babies for couples from all over the globe (Williams and Kress 2012). In my own interviews with doctors I found that the numbers varied widely, with different clinics reporting 10 to 70 women pregnant at any given time. Yet these numbers only count women who are currently pregnant and do not include the large number of women who approach doctors to become surrogates, undergo the medical procedures, and do not become pregnant or have miscarriages early in the pregnancy. Indeed, agents I spoke with indicated that more and more women, perhaps in the hundreds, were approaching them to learn about becoming surrogates or egg donors.

The screening process subjects surrogates to a battery of medical tests that must show they are healthy and free of disease. In addition, some clinics require a screening with the staff psychologist who can attest to the surrogates' emotional health and well-being. Most clinics require surrogates to be married with at least one but fewer than four children.[5] In general, surrogate recruitment patterns reflected a pyramid of sorts: women (typically former surrogates or egg donors) would recruit women in their communities whom they would then bring to another agent who conducted screenings and arranged payments, among other tasks. This higher-level agent, who acted as a broker between the local agents and the surrogacy clinics, would send surrogates to different agencies and clinics with whom she worked.

Once the intended parents select a clinic (or a medical tourism agency that acts as a go-between among the clients and the Indian agency or clinic), they may also face the decision of how to select an egg donor, if they are a gay male couple or an infertile married couple in which the intended mother cannot produce viable eggs. In general, parents who sought to minimize their costs and did not feel strongly about having a child with a particular phenotype would choose to select a donor from within India, usually through the same agency they were using for surrogacy. Others could choose to fly in an egg donor from another country; in this case, intended parents might choose to go with a clinic that already had a working relationship with their Indian surrogacy agency, or they might find their donor independently through a global egg donor agency. Some prospective parents bring an egg donor to India, typically a relative or friend who provides the egg for free.

When a couple has committed to a particular agency, they plan their first trip to India where they will meet their doctors, and in some cases the surrogate, for the first time. During this first trip, they will typically tour the facilities and meet key actors; many clients plan additional side trips for tourism purposes. They will also sign contracts at this stage, though not always in the company of the surrogate, who may sign the contract at a later date. In most cases I encountered, surrogacy contracts bind the couple and the surrogate, but the clinic rarely enters into this agreement. Prior to the 2015 ban on surrogacy services for foreigners, surrogacy was considered legal for foreigners in India, though no law regulated it and some doctors claimed that the contracts were not legally binding.

According to surrogates in this study, contract procedures were often opaque. Contracts are typically written in English, so a doctor or lawyer explains its contents to the surrogate. However, many surrogates reported receiving only cursory explanations of its contents, while others were simply instructed where to sign. In general, the contracts included no stipulations regarding payment; their main goal was to establish the parentage of the commissioning parents and to ensure that the surrogate would not attempt to prevent the parents from collecting their baby. Most clinics require surrogates' husbands to sign affidavits indicating their understanding of and agreement to their wife's surrogacy. If the surrogate is not married or no husband is present, then a parent or other relative of the surrogate must sign the affidavit.

In contrast to surrogacy in other countries, treatment in India often begins before the contract is signed. Because parents often have a limited amount of time to spend in India, they must begin the treatment protocols before they even land in India. If fresh embryos are to be used, the surrogate and the intended mother's or egg donor's menstrual cycles must be synchronized: the surrogate receives hormones in injections or pills while the intended mother or donor administers daily hormonal injections to stimulate her ovaries. These treatments must be timed so that multiple eggs will mature in one cycle and be ready for extraction when the surrogate's uterine lining reaches optimum thickness. The ova are then extracted and fertilized through IVF in a petri dish with the intended father's sperm; the resultant embryos are then transferred into the surrogate's uterus within forty-eight hours.

In some cases frozen embryos are used, in which case only the surrogate's body is monitored. Clients often choose to freeze embryos when they have "leftover" embryos from previous attempts. If their first attempt did not result in pregnancy, they can turn to frozen embryos (and avoid the hassle of planning additional trips to India). In other cases, clients may choose to work with agencies that facilitate the shipment of sperm, eggs, and embryos to India so that they do not have to travel until the birth of their child.

If the surrogate becomes pregnant, she continues to take hormonal medications for approximately the first twelve weeks of pregnancy, at which point her body "takes over" the pregnancy. During the pregnancy, she may move with her family to another apartment (organized by the agency), live in a home with surrogates away from her family, or remain in her community. Depending on the clinic, she may have an opportunity to meet the intended parents, or the parties may remain completely anonymous throughout the process. If clinics do encourage communication, much of the contact is by phone or Skype and mediated by clinic personnel who act as translators. If they do meet face-to-face before the birth, the meeting is often brief.

Parents normally plan their return trip to coincide with the due date of the child. They often plan longer stays in India at this time, to account for possible delays in processing paperwork and acquiring the travel documents necessary to return home with the child. At the time of my research, many (though not all) surrogacy babies were born at one particular hospital in Mumbai in which it was known that doctors would record the commissioning parents' names, not the surrogate's, on the birth certificate, which facilitated the process of obtaining the newborn's travel documents. Once the baby is born, the parents and surrogate may meet once—most parents described this as meeting "by accident"—but typically they do not maintain contact. In some cases parents may require further assistance from the surrogate as they plan their departure from India; some countries, such as Norway, require that the birth mother formally declare her intention to hand over the baby to the clients in order to obtain citizenship and travel documents for the child to return home.

Clearly, these stages and structures of transnational surrogacy require a complex coordination of multiple actors in the conception of a child; notwithstanding this complicated process of conception, the surrogacy industry thrived in India. In the final section of this chapter, I will briefly discuss the range of surrogacy practices I encountered in India, describing key aspects and differences in surrogacy practices among the clinics included in this research.

Contrasting Practices of Surrogacy

Karishma, whose story of providing donor eggs and gestational surrogacy I discussed at the beginning of this chapter, exemplified an evolving understanding of the role of people such as herself in transnational surrogacy. Her feelings about Dr. Singh changed over the time I knew her. Reflecting on her experience signing her contract, Karishma explained,

> Dr. Singh changes the contracts every year. She rushed and finished my contract signing in December. I don't feel like going back to her [as a surrogate] now or in the future. Everywhere they change the contracts because the amount increases every year. She did not tell me this and rushed it in December. She did not tell me that there would be an increase in payment if it was signed in January of this year. I learned about this later and now I don't want to go back to Dr. Singh. My contract was signed for U.S.$3,800 while this year surrogates get U.S.$5,500. Dr. Singh did not explain this to me; the other women who went to Dr. Singh and signed the surrogacy contract in January 2010 told me.

At the time of my research in India, doctors largely had the freedom to conduct their practices as they wished. Unfortunately, as Karishma found, this had an adverse impact for women who were uninformed or had little bargaining power when it came to their earnings as surrogates.

As discussed above, clinic practices tend to follow similar sequences and structures, yet their surrogacy practices may vary widely, offering a range of options to consumers of ARTs. Through my observation in a wide range of clinics and interviews with doctors, intended parents, surrogates, agents, and egg donors, I was able to gain various perspectives on different clinics and their surrogacy practices. The primary differences among clinics I encountered fall under the following categories:

Criteria for accepting clients—As one surrogacy doctor, Dr. Guha, explained to me, "We are giving birth to a non-existing child, we are giving a life to that baby, which never would have been there otherwise. That's why we screen our parents very strictly." Doctors' criteria for accepting clients reflected their own ideas and that of their culture about the kind of people they considered "appropriate" parents with respect to age, marital status, sexual orientation, and income. Dr. Guha's clinic, for example, accepted gay couples, married heterosexual couples, and single intended parents. His agency also required documentation such as bank statements and proof of home residence, noting, "It's our way of saying you have to have funds in the bank and you can't pay for this in credit." Other clinics refuse gay couples and single people. Some doctors imposed age limits—typically forty-five. One doctor told me that older parents would not be able to give a child a "proper life." Other doctors were known for accepting intended parents in their fifties and sixties. These criteria also revealed many doctors' belief in their responsibility as gatekeepers in the making of families. Dr. Guha, for instance, strongly believed he had great power to determine what sorts of families should be made: "Here we have a role to play. Here we are creating that baby."

Treatment and care of surrogates—Treatment and care of surrogates varied widely among clinics, particularly with respect to housing. While some doctors request that surrogates move to different accommodations with their families, others ask them to move to housing by themselves to live with other surrogates. Still others remain at home with their families in their communities for the duration of their pregnancies. Doctors expressed different rationales for these policies. On the one hand, doctors claimed that moving surrogates to new housing without their families allowed them to focus on taking care of themselves during pregnancy, without having to worry about work or family responsibilities. Others argued that in order for women to remain as psychologically and emotionally healthy as possible, surrogates must remain with their families. Some required women to move their families only if their family residence was inconvenient to the hospital. Some intended parents were sensitive to this issue, either preferring to know that the surrogate wouldn't be separated from her home, or alternatively that the surrogate would be closely monitored throughout pregnancy.

Management of relations between parents and surrogates—Communication between surrogates and parents was another area in which doctors held diverse views. Some clinics insist that parents and surrogates must not communicate at all during the course of the pregnancy and believe that an anonymous relationship is in the best interests of the parties involved. Doctors who had a significant number of gay clients often cited the stigma of homosexuality in India as a reason for barring communication, although my interviewees generally said they had no issues with gay parenting. Others expressed concern that surrogates might exploit the parents by asking for money or other aid. Other doctors encouraged contact, saying that it created strong bonds and relationships between parents and surrogates, thus improving the surrogacy experience for all involved. I also found that doctors' policies did not always dictate practice, and many who frowned on communication between surrogates and intended parents would facilitate online meetings when intended parents insisted. Some intended parents said that distance from the surrogates was an advantage of surrogacy in India.

Contracts and payment—I found that contract practices and payment plans varied widely among doctors. With no laws regulating the practice, doctors decided how to structure their own payment plans. Surrogates in this study said they earned a base rate of approximately U.S.$4,400 to U.S.$5,500. They received an additional U.S.$550–650 for carrying twins and U.S.$1,000–1,700 for undergoing cesarean section. One doctor in Delhi said he paid surrogates an additional U.S.$2,500–3,000 for enduring cesarean surgery. Doctors and surrogates made contradictory reports to me as to how much surrogates received. Some doctors offered extra payments for twin pregnancies or cesarean section births, but as one doctor told me, some felt that "a pregnancy is a pregnancy."

Doctors' charges for medical treatments and other services also varied widely, and as commissioning parents made inquiries to varied clinics across the country, they reported that doctors' fees were a major factor in their decisions about which clinic to attend. Parents typically paid at least five times what surrogates received and believed that surrogates received higher payments than the surrogates described. One Mumbai clinic, for example, charged more than U.S.$5,000 for registration, administrative costs, and costs associated with the surrogate's medical treatments (including preparation, embryo transfer, and prenatal care). The clinic charged another U.S.$6,600 for costs related to IVF (including medications), and this number rose to U.S.$11,500 if donor eggs were used. Thus, in one clinic fees for administrative and medical costs alone could range from U.S.$12,300 to U.S.$17,200. The same clinic charged parents approximately U.S.$2,200 for surrogate housing, and U.S.$2,200 for payments to the social worker, recruiter, and/or surrogate caretaker. In contrast, parents who attended other clinics reported paying substantially smaller package fees (for medical treatment, surrogate payments, and housing, among other costs). Thus, total payments to clinics for surrogacy services could range from U.S.$20,000 to U.S.$35,000.

Each of the clinic practices discussed above illustrates the diverse ways in which clinics, parents, and surrogates engage in commercial gestational surrogacy in the absence of any binding regulations. These practices also profoundly impact the ways in which actors experience surrogacy. In this research, I noted that several key themes emerged as a consequence of these practices, particularly with respect to kinship (as actors attempt to develop, or not, relationships with each other), race (as actors' ideas about kinship often intersect with particular constructions of race), and agency (as women attempt to navigate and negotiate payments, contracts, and medical treatments throughout their pregnancies). I suggest that the particular structures and practices of transnational surrogacy in India give salience to these themes, which are the focus of the chapters to follow.

This chapter situates Indian transnational surrogacy in relation to a broader context of public health, assisted reproduction, and medical tourism in India. I have demonstrated how assisted reproduction emerged in the context of neoliberalism, as public health approaches that focused on free comprehensive primary health care shifted to prioritize privatized health care services. These shifts occurred in a legal vacuum in which no laws existed regulating surrogacy or ARTs. India, then, was well situated to become a global destination for reproductive tourism in the early years of the twenty-first century. Thus, as the transnational surrogacy industry grew, the range of contexts and practices of surrogacy diverged in multiple directions, each imbricated in structures of inequality. The following chapters examine the various ways in which transnational surrogacy maintains and reinforces local and global structures of stratification.

2

Making Kinship, Othering Women

Surrogacy India, an agency dedicated to facilitating gestational surrogacy arrangements between Indian surrogates, egg donors, and a largely
international client base of would-be parents, earnestly offers an uncon-
ventional route to parenthood. One of the first to market their services
to foreign clients as the Indian surrogacy industry expanded starting
in 2005, today Surrogacy India is one of numerous agencies providing
surrogacy packages to infertile couples and individuals from around the
world. The agency justifies the promise of IVF and gestational surrogacy
by emphasizing genetic models of kinship: "To reproduce is the strongest human desire, second only to survival itself. If none of us passed on
our DNA and refuse [*sic*] to become parents, life would end with us."[1]
The use of such affective language to highlight primordial desires for
biogenetically related children was not unusual among Indian doctors
in their efforts to draw prospective clients to their clinics and to situate
their own ethical and moral positions regarding surrogacy. Indeed, as
one doctor explained, "Every human being has the right to be a parent.
Who are we to decide who should and cannot? Surrogacy is not a crime.
It is an alternative mode of delivery for all those who are interested in
having their own biological children." To be sure, by and large doctors
argued that couples seek gestational surrogacy because of a desire for
their "own child," and surrogates, egg donors, and commissioning parents frequently embraced claims to parenthood as an inalienable right
and a desire innate to human beings.

Yet the unique circumstances of family making via transnational gestational surrogacy in India call into question dominant ideas of kinship and parenthood among the range of actors involved, and rely on
multiple disruptive boundary crossings. Consumers of transnational
surrogacy in India travel across national boundaries in order to hire
surrogate mothers, often of a racial background different than their
own. Indeed, Surrogacy India's home page boasts a series of cartoons

that portray the "typical" actors involved in transnational surrogacy, unambiguously highlighting differences in class, nation, and culture. The commissioning parents appear as a conventional white Western married couple, with the husband dressed in a shirt and tie and the wife in high heels and a knee-length skirt, her haircut stylishly short. The surrogate mother, meanwhile, is sketched as a stereotypical "traditional" Indian woman; she is visibly pregnant with her long hair in a bun, wearing a *dupatta* over her housedress and a *bindi* on her forehead. The images and discourse found throughout the website emphasize the creation of perfect (white) children and the making of happy (white) families. Moreover, these illustrations center on and naturalize difference and distance between Western commissioning parents and Indian surrogates. Indeed, themes in the agency's promotional materials explicitly code the Indian woman as racially and culturally Other to the commissioning parents as well as to the fetus she bears. As Surrogacy India's pamphlets state, India represents the ideal global destination for gestational surrogacy, in part because "Indian culture is much different from the rest of the world. No Indian woman has the desire to carry your Caucasian [or other raced] children in her arms as she would not be able to explain or bear the social stigma."[2]

Clearly, transnational surrogacy in India underlines the intersection of ideas about kinship, genetics, race, and reproduction. The readiness of primarily white, Western commissioning parents to enlist Indian women in gestational surrogacy arrangements can be traced in part to the belief in popular scientific discourse that compartmentalizes gestation and genetics. That is, if the qualities that determine a child's future identity are embedded in his or her genes, then the role and influence of the gestational surrogate matters less, because she makes no genetic contribution (even though she undoubtedly shares a biological connection to the child because of the embodied nature of surrogacy). Yet this genetic essentialism—the notion that human beings can be reduced to their genes, privileging genetics over gestation in the context of assisted reproduction—raises questions about how actors construct kinship, race, and racial difference. In other words, how do commissioning parents, doctors, and others conceive of the connections between racial identity, genetic reproduction, and cultural attitudes about kinship and relatedness?

In this chapter, I examine the ways in which intended parents understand kinship and parenthood as they narrate their family's origin stories, as well as how these constructions of kinship intersect with specific racial formations. I found that infertile couples and individuals who pursue surrogacy in India employ a range of strategies to create and make sense of their connections with surrogates, egg donors, and children conceived through gestational surrogacy, where biogenetic and social kinship ties are alternately challenged, transformed, or reinforced. These kinship narratives, I argue, frequently intersect with processes of Othering that allow parents to view the nation of India and Indian women as fundamentally different. I demonstrate the ways in which commissioning parents construct notions of race within their family's origin stories, as they emphasize implied racial difference in order to view Indian women alternately as objects of rescue or as manipulative actors solely concerned with financial remuneration. By examining the ways in which would-be parents engage with medical models of kinship and racialized constructions of surrogates to create their own familial "origin" stories, I illuminate the ways in which commissioning parents naturalize hierarchies of difference embedded in surrogacy in India. In other words, analyzing the ways in which ideologies of kinship and race coproduce one another reveals the strategies actors use to justify surrogacy arrangements that are fraught with inequality.

By contextualizing participants' comments in a discussion of current and historical discourses about biogenetic connections, race, and kinship, I show how various actors think about these themes when making decisions about building their own families. For example, nearly 90 percent of intended parents interviewed mentioned at some point the importance of genetics in the process of conception. Yet they also expressed variable views about the significance of genes vis-à-vis their own relationship to the child. While the concept of "lineage" emerged throughout many conversations with intended parents, few used it as a justification for traveling to India for surrogacy. Indeed, throughout my interviews with 39 intended parents, only 9 (or 23 percent) explicitly mentioned their desire for a genetically related child as a motivating reason for traveling to India for surrogacy. Instead, intended parents articulated a wide range of ideas and beliefs about parenthood and kinship, which were deeply informed by hierarchies of race, nationality, and class. I focus on the ways in which biogenetic relationships and particular racial imaginaries figured into informants' narratives, illuminating how actors build, create, or deny kinship bonds with one another, as well as with the child born via gestational surrogacy. Building on the work of anthropologists who have shown how transracial and international adoption challenges inherited understandings of identity, kinship, and belonging (Gailey 2010; Yngvesson 2010), I suggest that transnational surrogacy creates global relationships across race and nation that challenge existing notions of kinship in creative and meaningful ways.

In particular, I argue that commissioning parents' kinship narratives hinge on two kinds of racial imaginaries. On the one hand, parents' surrogacy stories often constructed the Indian surrogate as an object of rescue, intertwining narratives of their families' origins with narratives of rescue or the empowerment of Indian women. Uneven relations of class, race, and nation were a source of tension among many intended parents uncomfortable with the commercial aspects of surrogacy, and they employed various strategies to resolve these tensions. In particular, commissioning parents utilized rescue narratives that describe surrogacy as a "win-win situation," in which they gain a child while providing an income to a woman in need. As one U.S. father of three children born through surrogacy in India stated, "With an Indian surrogate, you are fundamentally changing the trajectory of her life." Indeed, many parents justify the remarkable nature of their kinship stories through the humanitarian aspects implicated in transnational surrogacy—the promise of profoundly improving the lives of poor Indian women. Such narratives, however, invoke essentialized, one-dimensional portraits of the surrogate as a saint or mother, and position the Western family as saving the Indian surrogate, making the woman herself a humanitarian object (an identity that relies on her role as a mother to her own children). I suggest that commissioning parents rely on constructions of the Indian surrogate as racially Other to Western clients and their families in order to make the Indian surrogate worthy of saving.

On the other hand, not all the parents I spoke with resorted to narratives of rescue as a strategy to resolve the anxieties related to commercial surrogacy. Indeed, about a third of intended parents expressed their deep suspicion of what one called a "hero myth" and confronted the commodifying features of family making in distinct ways, often describing surrogacy as explicitly transactional—nothing more than a business deal in which the client pays the surrogate for her reproductive labor. In this context, rather than view the Indian surrogate as an object to be rescued, clients depict the surrogate as a worker doing a job, one that is detached from emotional labor. This depiction consequently translates into the portrayal of commercial surrogates as cold-hearted and easily able to renounce the child that they carry (see also Teman 2008). Often the surrogate is constructed as a figure of suspicion; she is cast as a potentially shrewd manipulator, cunningly working to extract undeserved remuneration from unsuspecting parents-to-be. This figure of the surrogate as a potential threat, similar to that of the surrogate as an object to be rescued, possesses an implicit racialization, one that establishes the population of surrogate women as racially Other and nonwhite. As I will discuss, even when parents eschew notions of rescue and view surrogacy as clearly transactional, emphasizing the remuneration that surrogates receive, their narratives nonetheless reinforce imbalances of power between surrogates and parents.

Kinship, Race, and Rescue

Previous ethnographies of surrogacy have elucidated the role of the "gift narrative" as a cultural tool for justifying family making through gestational surrogacy. Indeed, for many intended parents, the practice of "kinning," or the process by which parents, children, and surrogates are made into kin,[3] relies on gift narratives as a strategy for rendering more palatable the discomfiting commercial aspects of surrogacy. As Marilyn Strathern writes in her analysis of organ and tissue donation, "The language of the gift conceals commodification of the body" (2012, 401), and in the context of commercial surrogacy the language of the gift takes several forms. In her study of surrogacy in the United States, for instance, Helena Ragoné demonstrates the ways in which surrogates deemphasized receiving remuneration and instead highlighted their motivation to give "the ultimate gift of love" (1994, 59).

On the other hand, while anthropologist Elly Teman (2010) found that Israeli surrogates openly voiced their motives as mainly financial, they too depend on a gift rhetoric during the surrogacy process. Unlike in the United States, the Israeli surrogate does not offer the gift of a child; rather she sees herself as providing the gift of motherhood to another woman with whom she has developed a sisterly bond or close relationship. In doing so, Teman elucidates how surrogates and intended mothers become connected and "'shift' the pregnant body between them" (2010, 284), highlighting the ways in which surrogates detach, distance, and disembody aspects of pregnancy so that the intended mother may construct her own "pregnant identity." Surrogates simultaneously narrate their own surrogacy processes as a hero's journey, portraying themselves as courageous, mythic heroines, women who endure hardships in order to achieve increased self-knowledge, self-worth, and empowerment. Embedded in the "hero's quest" is the surrogates' "mission," in which their true goals include making a family and making an intended mother a real mother (2010, 264). Teman notes that paradoxically, however, surrogates embark on this sacred quest "within a highly structured framework that, arguably, represents the height of medicalization, commodification, and patriarchal institutional control of women's bodies" (2010, 277).

The gift narrative also finds traction in Indian surrogacy, though in unexpected ways. In her study of Indian surrogates in Garv, a city in western India, Pande (2014a) found that surrogates and intended mothers alike use discursive tools and narratives such as "global sisterhood," "gift of God," and "mission" to mask the transactional nature of commercial baby making. Intended mothers from the global North envision their travel for gestational surrogacy arrangements as a "mission"; here, what matters is their role in mitigating the effects of poverty and saving a "worthy" Indian family. As Pande argues, the language of mission reifies the inequities of race, class, and nationality on which transnational surrogacy is based.

Interestingly, the gift narrative found less traction among commissioning parents in my study. Instead, ideologies of rescue, aid, and humanitarianism more powerfully evoked the attitudes of would-be parents. Here, actors construct transnational surrogacy as a form of humanitarian aid or as a duty of socially conscious citizens, and such narratives of rescue are intertwined with particular racial imaginaries. In this context, scholarship on transnational and transracial adoption offers an important framework for understanding the intersection of rescue narratives, race, and kinship.

Intended parents' ways of describing their relationship to the surrogate that would bring their children into the world participate in a tradition of narratives of rescue that extend backward to colonialism.[4] These historically influential scripts continue to resonate in the twenty-first century, though the objects of rescue are distinct, as are the social contexts in which the rescue narratives unfold. More recently, scholars have explicated how rescue narratives emerge in the context of transnational adoption, with questions of belonging, race, and culture looming large. Eng (2003), for instance, describes the original "humanitarian" justifications for transnational adoption, particularly after World War II when overseas adoption began to take hold in the United States. Examining the ways in which the adopted child is both object and subject, Eng demonstrates how transnational adoption reproduces the white heterosexual nuclear family. In other words, whiteness, the American family, and nation are enacted through the transnational adoptee's racial and cultural difference (Ortiz and Briggs 2003).

Yet while the consumption of exotic difference reproduces hegemonic forms of family and nation, the vulnerability and marginalization of children emerges as one of the most desirable kinds of difference. Patton elucidates the ways in which "the 1960s impetus toward the placement of 'hard-to-place' children—most prominently children of color—drew on racialized stories of salvation and rescue" (2000, 57). These stories, as Dorow suggests, "symbolically mitigated White privilege while simultaneously reproducing it under the guise of the 'good White liberal'" (2006, 363).

In China, agencies narrate the adoption of baby girls as a way to "rescue" them from a supposedly sexist culture. As Anagnost (2000) writes, the "theme of salvage" permeates many adoption narratives, in which the saving of the child is depicted as a heroic act. Ann Anagnost has analyzed rescue narratives in transnational adoption as "rituals of decommodification" which transform the commercial transaction into a sentimental possession that must be kept separate from the impersonal contract of market exchange. Such rituals of decommodification exist in transnational surrogacy too, yet parents confront the commodifying features of family making in distinct ways.

In transnational surrogacy, commissioning parents do not speak of saving children—only the surrogate mother. Surrogacy rescues women from poverty as well as from more distasteful work alternatives such as sex work, factory work, or poorly paid domestic work. Doctors in particular would frequently argue that surrogacy is a "win-win" situation that provides an income for a woman without having to resort to sex work, adding a moral spin to justifications of surrogacy and demonstrating the various imagined political economies that proliferate through surrogacy. Moreover, humanitarian justifications efface the need to acquire any in-depth knowledge of history, language, politics, and culture while masking the structural factors that motivate women to become surrogates. What counts in the rescue script is simply a desire to "help" women change their lives while simultaneously building their own families. Yet such language veils the fact that parents are not making charitable donations; they are paying women to carry out the labor of gestation and childbirth.

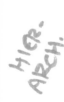

Moreover, these rescue scripts rely on the construction of racial imaginaries that Other surrogates in order to justify their rescue. DasGupta and Dasgupta have previously shown how race functions to Other Indian gestational surrogates from the fetus they carry, arguing that the practices of Othering surrogates and India themselves operate as a "cybernetic imperialist discourse," which position the surrogate as one minor player among many in the process of transnational baby making (2014b, 82). I go further to connect these processes of Othering to specific practices that enable commissioning parents to view Indian women alternately as objects to be rescued or as women solely concerned with remuneration. Each of these constructions relies on a particular racial imaginary of the surrogate. On the one hand, commissioning parents use language that masks the commercial transaction that brings about the life of their child and makes surrogacy about "saving" women from poverty or "empowering" them to help their own families. On the other, parents-to-be construct Indian women as mere reproductive workers or as potentially shrewd manipulators whose sole motivation is remuneration. In both cases, Indian surrogates are implicitly marked as a population of racial Others. In doing so, transnational surrogacy brings people together in the name of family making while simultaneously masking inequalities of class and nationality.

The Epitome of Motherhood

I first met Adam and Nadine in the waiting room of Origins Gynecology Clinic, a busy infertility clinic in South Mumbai. At the time of our interview, Nadine and Adam were forty-three and forty-seven years old, respectively, and they had recently celebrated twenty-five years together, having met when Nadine was eighteen. Six years prior to our meeting in Mumbai, Nadine was diagnosed with stage three colon cancer; as a result, she endured rounds of chemotherapy that she says "burned her eggs," as well as a hysterectomy. Once she was declared "clear" of the cancer, Adam and Nadine decided to move forward with their desire to have children. They looked first at adoption—the first logical step, in their minds—and were immediately turned off by the process, which they found to be invasive and discriminatory. Based in Texas, Adam and Nadine found that many adoption agencies were Christian; staunch atheists, they were horrified when an adoption consultant told them it was OK that they weren't Christian, "as long as you've never set foot in a synagogue in the past." Moreover, the racial politics involved in adoption bothered Adam and Nadine, who were both white. As Nadine recalled, "The adoption consultant asked, 'How quick do you want a baby? Do you want a white baby? A half-white baby? Do you want a Mexican baby? A half-Mexican baby? Do you want a black baby?' . . . And if you want a Caucasian baby, forget it. Nobody gets Caucasian babies." "As if you could just grab one off the shelf," Adam interjected. "It was complete objectification."

They thought they might have to forgo having children when Adam saw a television special on surrogacy in India. He started to do some research and found that the costs of surrogacy in the United States were too prohibitive, so they chose to work with an agency in Australia that had a relationship with Origins Clinic in Mumbai. He learned that this agency also had ties with a clinic in South Africa, through which they would be able to select a white egg donor. Interestingly, while they appeared uncomfortable with making decisions about adoption based on ethnicity, when it came to assisted reproduction Adam and Nadine were clear about their preference for a white egg donor. According to Adam and Nadine, a child that resembled them phenotypically would not raise questions among strangers, allowing them to "control the dissemination of information" to their child about his or her origins. As they explained, "No one will ask, why are mommy and daddy a different color from you?" If the child were white, Adam and Nadine themselves could decide when and how they would disclose the story of how the child came into being.

Yet while Adam and Nadine took exception to the racialized structures that commodified child adoptees, they simultaneously accepted the commodification of donor gametes based on race and ethnicity, exercising their consumer power to select their preferred "white" donor eggs. Moreover, this explanation does not shed light on why Adam and Nadine's surrogacy process would be very different from adopting a white child, indicating, perhaps, an elaborate rationalization for pursuing surrogacy—and a child that would be genetically related to Adam. It also recalls what Becker et al. call "resemblance talk," or observations about a child's resemblance to family members in order to affirm the legitimacy of the parents who used donor gametes to conceive a child (Becker, Butler, and Nachtigall 2005). Yet as Becker and colleagues argue, comments about a child's resemblance to parents may make it more difficult, not easier, for parents to disclose the true nature of their child's conception as long as kinship models that privilege genetic connectedness prevail.

With all the arrangements made, Adam and Nadine embarked on a journey to India that they hoped would result in parenthood. However, as we talked about families and parenthood, it became clear that Adam and Nadine's own personal histories had played a major role in their imaginings of the other actors in surrogacy, especially the surrogate mother. Both Adam and Nadine spoke at length about how they each came from families with histories of abuse and neglect. Indeed, they confessed that their relationships with their own parents influenced their desire to delay having children until they were absolutely ready. This resulted in an explicit denial of the importance of biology in defining kinship or relatedness. As Nadine observed, "For me, having grown up with a mother who was abusive and neglectful, I definitely don't have the idea that the person biologically related to you is the best person to be your mother. That person can often be the worst person to be your mother." She went on to explain, "It's not the blood ties; it's the emotional ties that connect you. It's the emotional ties that connect us to the people we love and care about." Adam agreed: "You're talking to two people who don't put a lot of stock in biology. . . . Being a mom is not about delivering an egg and being a dad is not about delivering sperm. It's like—and I hate to sound a little clichéd—but it's every day, for the rest of the child's life and your life. . . . The thing is, the minute that child can breathe that first breath on their own, parenting starts."

While Adam and Nadine preferred a child that resembled them racially, they simultaneously deemphasized the importance of biogenetic relatedness in favor of parenthood models that emphasized social, nurturing roles. Similarly, Helena Ragoné's (1996) study of surrogacy in the United States illustrates how both commissioning couples and surrogates deemphasize biogenetic connections in order to highlight the importance of social parenthood. In doing so, they collaboratively reinterpret motherhood as primarily social, emphasizing the adoptive mother's nurturant role in order to dodge questions of biogenetic origins. Such ideologies of motherhood that rely on the relationship of caring, however, inevitably contain contradictions. Analyzing the famous surrogacy case of Baby M, Barbara Katz Rothman has argued that if paternity and maternity depended on the social relationship of caring, then the connection the pregnant women form while carrying a fetus for nine months would cement their rights as mothers (Rothman 1989).

Indeed, as we were discussing motherhood, Nadine confided, "I think that there's this beautiful idea of the mother who begins nurturing and caring for that baby when it's still a fetus. She begins teaching it, right from the beginning, by the way they're putting different food in their body." As Nadine was preparing to raise a child that would not be genetically related to her, she asserted that biological relatedness was not what defined parenthood. Yet at the same time she could not deny the bond that exists between a mother and the fetus growing inside her. Nadine went on to contextualize their decision to pursue surrogacy in India:

Surrogacy seemed right in India. Women here, they need the money. The doctors were saying they were going to use the money to put their kids in school; it's always for their children, their future. *And talk about a mom—that's the epitome of motherhood.* That this woman is willing to carry someone else's baby inside of her! For nine months! That is an act of selflessness, because she's doing it for her children, to improve the future of her children. *I want to be half that mom. And I would be an incredible mom if I were half that mom.* [emphasis in the original]

Nadine's comments reveal the complexities and contradictions inherent in gestational surrogacy as well as in the meanings she attached to motherhood. In the context of surrogacy, Nadine's understanding of her own and the surrogate mother's relationship to the child born through surrogacy simultaneously affirm and deny biological motherhood, offering a powerful lesson in how unsettled are the debates on nature versus nurture.

Nadine's narrative also reflects a common theme among many intended parents I met, where the surrogate's own role as a birth mother to surrogate babies might be deemphasized while elevating her role as a mother to her own children. Indeed, many women spoke admiringly of their surrogates and their devotion to their children. As Nadine noted, women form an intimate bond with the fetus through gestational surrogacy, yet in order to affirm Nadine's role as the mother the surrogate's kinship with the child must be deemphasized by highlighting her motherhood to her own children. Nadine achieved this by highlighting the surrogate's "need" and her desire to "improve the future of her own children." This discursive move simultaneously shifted the focus from commodification to rescue, while locating motherhood squarely within the surrogate's own family (denying any possibility of motherhood to the fetus the surrogate carries). At the same time, Nadine Othered Indian women by expressing a romanticized and potentially colonizing notion of Indian identity, as her remarks echo the justifications offered by many Indian doctors for India's emergence as a global hub for surrogacy. Dr. Nayna Patel, for instance, hinted at the importance that Hinduism places on childbearing and parenthood, as well as the prospect of being rewarded in the next life for good deeds in this one, in order to explain Indian women's enthusiasm and why they were suitable for surrogacy (Chu 2006).

Indeed, Nadine's comments appear to reinforce ideologies of Indian motherhood. In India, motherhood is traditionally considered nearly divine and central to a women's gender identity and the essence of femininity (Hegde 1999; Jain 2003; Krishnaraj 2010). Within Indian societies, women fulfill their nurturing and ideal role only when they become mothers and motherhood remains the primary *raison d'etre* of most Indian women (Nandy 1976; Wadley 1977). Indeed, in a study of sex workers in Kolkata, the majority of women in the sex trade argued that motherhood was their primary purpose in life (Sinha and Dasgupta 2009).

Yet, as DasGupta and Dasgupta argue, gestational surrogacy jeopardizes traditional constructions of Indian motherhood, as "Indian women become reduced to their body parts at the sacrifice of their most empowered social role" (2010, 146). Indeed, Nadine's narrative reflects the many contradictions at the intersection of motherhood and transnational surrogacy. Even as Nadine underscored the surrogate's role as a mother to her own children and as a nurturer of the fetus she was carrying, global surrogacy arrangements privilege Western parenthood over Indian motherhood. Indeed, surrogacy often separated women from their own children when doctors required surrogates to live in housing closer to the hospital. To be sure, doctors often claimed that they provided better housing for surrogates and their families during the course of their pregnancies. In my observation, however, the housing resembled the one-room apartments women rented with their families, although the location took women from their husbands, whose jobs kept them home, and from their extended families. Women who couldn't or wouldn't be separated from their children had to remove their children from school. Commissioning parents like Adam and Nadine were ignorant of all this.

Despite Adam and Nadine's desire to know their child's surrogate and to express their gratitude to her, Nadine found their first and only meeting with the surrogate deeply disappointing. As the couple arrived at the agency office to sign their contracts, they expected to meet only the lawyer. Yet when they arrived, they learned that their surrogate and her friend were already there. Instantly feeling awkward, hopeful, unprepared, and excited, Adam and Nadine waited for an opportunity to be introduced to the woman who would carry their child. Instead, agency staff bluntly asked the couple, "Do you want her to go?" Adam and Nadine found the question strange, interpreting it as if the staff was asking whether they required the surrogate to leave. "Of course," Nadine told me, "we would have said we would love it if *she* would like to stay," but, bewildered, the couple hesitated. Adam noticed that she was sitting in the waiting room and thought with relief that she would stay; then, he says, "The next time I looked up after signing the contract, she was gone."

Adam and Nadine attributed the awkwardness of this encounter, in which they never formally met or exchanged words with their surrogate, to the hierarchies of class. Nadine recalled, "She's doing something amazing for us and I wanted to at least show her some sort of gratitude, some sort of civility, and it didn't seem like it was very civil. I don't know if that's because of her social status, in relation to the lawyer. It's hard to tell because everyone is so poor." Adam and Nadine felt deeply conflicted about the hierarchies of nationality and class that permeated their relationship with the surrogate and expressed profound disappointment with the way the doctors and lawyers mediated their communication with her.

"A Variation on the Theme of Your Life": Orientalist Narratives and Racial Distancing

While Adam and Nadine did not strongly desire a genetically related child, Diana felt otherwise. When I first met Diana on a rainy day during monsoon season, she was at the start of her third visit to India within a year. Born in Europe but a resident of the United States for more than a decade, she was in the midst of receiving hormone injections to stimulate the production of ovarian follicles in anticipation of her upcoming egg retrieval procedure. Diana's extracted eggs would be fertilized with her husband's sperm, and the resulting embryos would then be transferred to an Indian woman. Diana's previous two attempts at surrogacy in Mumbai did not result in pregnancy, and while she acknowledged the emotional and physical strain of the surrogacy process on both herself and her husband, Lenny, Diana's desire for a genetically related child was strong, and she maintained a positive outlook and embraced her travels to India as part of a grand adventure.

At the time of our interview, Diana was a successful media professional in her early forties. She had met and married her husband several years earlier, and after initial attempts to start a family Diana learned that she had very large uterine fibroids. Diana's doctors told her that even with surgery she would have a very slim chance of being able to carry a pregnancy to term. Shattered and overwhelmed, it was at this point that Diana learned about surrogacy in India, just as she was contemplating adoption "with a heavy heart." I asked Diana why she viewed adoption in this way, and she responded:

> Adoption is a very different process. But the fact that you cannot extend your lineage any longer is a very difficult thing to come to terms with. Surrogacy, although it's quite complicated, and requires a lot of medication and a lot of legal things are involved and it's very costly—one thing that it definitely offers is the last opportunity to try to extend your lineage so you can actually have your own children. And a lot of people underestimate how important that is.

Diana was part of a minority of intended parents with whom I spoke who explicitly noted the importance of lineage, or having one's "own" children, in their surrogacy journeys. She was also unusual in using her own egg. Although Diana acknowledged the high costs, risks, and legal complexities associated with transnational surrogacy, she nonetheless argued that the imperative to parent one's own genetic offspring justified these obstacles. Yet while Diana argued that surrogacy offered a valid option for infertile parents seeking genetically related children, her comments also reveal the reality that surrogacy is an expensive, high-risk technology, sought after by infertile parents desperate for a "last opportunity" at parenthood and willing to overlook the reality of the low success rates of surrogacy.

I asked Diana if she could expand on the importance of carrying forth her lineage. After lamenting the bureaucratic difficulties of adoption and the anticipated restrictions due to her and Lenny's "advanced" ages, she replied,

> There is something to be said for having your own child. Absolutely. Because when the child comes from your own environment, inheriting your DNA, and something of your outlook on life, it's kind of like a variation on your theme of life. But if you adopt the child, then it's from a completely different part of the world and it's a completely different story. . . . Somehow I think that if it is *our* child, Lenny's and mine, then we're not only going to be influencing his life from the outside, but also from the

inside. From the fact that it is our flesh and blood. Well, just flesh, not blood; *the blood is going to be from the surrogate.* [emphasis added]

There are many tensions to be unpacked in Diana's comment. Interestingly, Diana explicitly drew a distinction between transnational adoption and transnational surrogacy; from her perspective, adoption entails incorporating into her family a child "from a completely different part of the world." Here, she emphasized difference; an adopted child would have a "different story," one in which Diana and Lenny would have little influence. Transnational surrogacy, on the other hand, allowed Diana to control the "story" and affect the child's life not only "from the outside, but also from the inside," reflecting the conventional wisdom that stresses the importance of genetic heritability (over social and environmental factors) in behavior and identity formation.

Moreover, Diana revealed the complexities involved in negotiating kinship in the context of gestational surrogacy. In contrast to Adam and Nadine, for Diana biogenetic connections were crucial in passing on "some variation of [their] theme of life." However, while Diana emphasized genetic connections, effectively Othering the surrogate from the fetus she carries, Diana simultaneously acknowledges that her surrogacy arrangement would not be possible without the surrogate's own blood. This was in contradiction to medical and policy language in India, which defines motherhood in terms of genetic or intended motherhood, effectively excluding the work of the gestational surrogate. Indeed, medical and policy documents consistently maintained that the legal parents of children born through surrogacy should be the commissioning couple or individual.

Diana's feelings about the importance of creating a son or daughter who was following up on the "theme" of her and her husband's life also challenges David Schneider's rendering of kinship in terms of substance: "relatives" are defined by "blood" and "[t]he blood relationship is thus a relationship of substance, of shared biogenetic material" (1980, 25). However, Schneider effectively equated blood and biogenetic substance; what the terms actually refer to has not always been clear (Carsten 2001, 2004). Indeed, many scholars have critiqued the essentialist and naturalized assumptions of kinship and substance, preferring to focus on the context of the relationships (Carsten 2000; Strathern

1992; Thompson 2005). Such works have shown how the boundaries between the social and the biological are "more permeable" in local discourses than was assumed by classic kinship studies (Carsten 2000, 10). Indeed, while it is recognized that mother and child share bodily substances like blood and breast milk, establishing automatic ties between mother and fetus, these shared substances do not trump the male contribution. As Fruzzetti and Östör (1984) explain in their study of kinship in Bengal, female bodily fluids may nourish the fetus but they do not confer identity on a child. Indeed, in the indigenous system of Ayurvedic medicine it is the male who contributes blood, as the child who inherits the father's seed also inherits his blood. In contrast, Indian surrogates in Pande's (2014c) study took a very different view of the blood tie, claiming that their blood not only sustains the fetus but also imparts an identity to the child. These ties manifest in what Pande calls "kin labor," or the range of labor surrogates perform in order to maintain their ties with the intended mother after birth, with other surrogates, and with the child itself.

Similarly, while Diana recognized the importance of the relationship between genetic parent and child, she also highlighted the role of the surrogate; indeed, it was the surrogate's blood that would nourish the child. When discussing the process of finding a surrogate in India, Diana expresses strong feelings about the importance of the surrogate's well-being:

> When I think about it, I want to make sure that my child is developed well, so the woman who is carrying him must be feeling good. I want her to feel happy when she's carrying this child. Because it's all connected. The fact that there is a word "surrogate" in front of the word "mother" does not change the fact that it's her emotions; it's her well-being that's going into the development of the child.

Diana's comments recall Jeanette Edwards's (1993) study of views of ARTs among residents of northwest England, specifically their opinions about what is transferred from mother to child through the placenta. Edwards's informants speculated that a baby nurtured in an artificial womb would lack a connection to its mother or her feelings. Similarly, while Adam and Nadine did not ascribe much importance to the role of genetics in their notion of parenthood, like Diana they highlighted the enduring impact of the surrogate and her relationship to the child.

But Diana acknowledged the stresses embedded in transnational surrogacy, particularly as intended parents engage in surrogacy arrangements characterized by profound socioeconomic inequality.

> It's very complicated. But, you know, in the end I just want to go through the process with my head held high. I've read so many articles where people are creating caricatures of the intended parents coming into the Third World country, taking advantage of the poor women. I've struggled with that quite a lot, I certainly have. I've felt like I've taken advantage of these poor women and yet I'm still going through it. And that was my big question for myself. Why is it I cannot stop and still must go through with it? And I guess it's the drive to have your own child. I don't know how else to explain it.

Here, Diana admitted her discomfort with the unequal relationships embedded in transnational surrogacy while simultaneously glossing over this tension to emphasize the drive to have one's "own child." In other words, Diana seemed to understand the ways in which surrogacy in India reflects what Boris and Parreñas (2010) call "intimate labor," or low-status "women's work" involving psychic and bodily intimacy, overwhelmingly performed by economically disadvantaged women. Yet in viewing the surrogate as a poor, Third World woman, Diana called attention to her "Third-World difference," described by Chandra Mohanty as "that stable, ahistorical something" that characterizes the lives of women in Third World countries as singular and monolithic (1988, 63). This contrasts with portrayals of Euro-American women who are complex, dynamic subjects; in Diana's case, women who grapple with the inequities embedded in transnational surrogacy arrangements but nonetheless prioritize their quests for a genetically related child.

Yet Diana felt strongly that if her current attempt resulted in a positive pregnancy, she would make every effort to return to India and spend time with her surrogate. Discussing the policy of several doctors to prohibit any relationship or communication between the intended parent and the surrogate, Diana responded, "I think that's very wrong. . . . I think that what they think they're doing is protecting the emotions of the parents and the surrogates. But what they're doing, in fact, is they're creating this alienation that everybody's afraid of." Diana had met the surrogate who had been implanted with her fertilized egg before, and she described a "very special connection" to her. Born in eastern Europe, she divulged that she "find[s] it easier to connect with Indian surrogate mothers" than American women. When I asked why, she replied:

> Because they have same basic values [as myself]. They are mothers, they are wives, they're family-oriented, they know what's like to have nothing and to share the little bit that they have. They have a good heart and for the most part they're not selfish. They do it of course to get the money, but underneath all that, I just find it easier to connect with them. I just happened to hear the story this morning about this gay couple who came to India to pick up their recent surrogate child; the first one was born to a surrogate in the United States, the second one was born to a surrogate in India. So they were telling stories how in the United States their surrogate's boyfriend was a drug addict, and they were constantly getting into trouble, constantly needing money, going into jail. It was like nonstop mayhem. So they had to take care of the surrogate and the boyfriend to make sure she can actually live through the experience and deliver the child that's semi-normal. Can you imagine! . . . Here you have a completely random stranger carrying your child that you cannot have by any other means. So you're really putting a lot of faith into this woman, and I think about the environment where they come from, and I think more about how their heart and the relationship that they have with their family, rather than how much money they have, will affect the process. I've been here three times already and I can honestly say that I feel much more comfortable with Indian surrogates.

Here, Diana explicitly positioned Indian surrogates against U.S. surrogates, aligning herself (with her eastern European background) with the Indian surrogates whom she constructed as having good values, being family-oriented, and not being selfish. Interestingly, her comments again recall conceptualizations of the surrogate in terms of

"Third-World difference," this time placing herself and the surrogate in contrast to U.S. women. But she simultaneously relied on the popular perception of India as a morally "pure" mystic East, in which Indian women avoid (Western) vices such as alcohol, smoking, and drugs. In contrast, surrogacy in the United States is deeply problematic, due in part to the surrogate's drug use, a problem she implied stems from Western culture and ideals. However, even though Diana's narrative depended on her own distancing from "the West," she relied on exotic frames that draw from Orientalist discourses of race and nation that construct "Indianness" as desirable *in relation* to the West, establishing Indian suitability for surrogacy as contingent upon being different enough from Western women and the West. Said (1978) and others have argued that "Asianness" necessitates no such comparison with the West but nonetheless is forced into one through Orientalist discourses.

Diana's comment also reflects an interesting twist on what Lisa Ikemoto (2009) calls "racial distancing." Discussing the ways in which mainstream media coverage represents the surrogacy business in India as exotic, highlighting racial, cultural, and economic differences, Ikemoto argues, "What these stories express is the persistence of a form of racial distancing that may make hiring a woman to gestate, give birth to, and give up a child psychologically comfortable. It is a post-industrial form of master-servant privilege. In effect, it makes the non-White woman in the non-White country a marketable source of surrogacy" (2009, 308). Indeed, Diana's comments illustrate the ways in which many intended parents racialize the Indian women involved in transnational surrogacy, relying on Orientalist frames and racial distancing to Other Indian surrogates.

Nobility and the Labor of Surrogacy

Aaron and Ben were thirty-eight and thirty-seven years old, respectively, when I first met them at their full-service apartment in a wealthy suburb of Mumbai. Israelis who had been together for eleven years, they had started taking steps toward having a family about six or seven years earlier when they first explored coparenting options with a single lesbian friend. Over six months, they discussed what having children together might entail, how the child would be educated, and where they would live. "It was a long process," Aaron explained, and eventually the three drew up a contract and started trying to have a baby. After several attempts, their friend became pregnant, but then miscarried in the first trimester.

Traumatized by the miscarriage, their friend eventually decided to back out of the deal and Aaron and Ben turned next to adoption. However, they found adoption in Israel to be nearly impossible due to the small number of available adoptees, and international adoption posed too many restrictions for gay couples. Aaron and Ben eventually decided on surrogacy abroad. As Israel prohibits gay couples from engaging in surrogacy and surrogacy in the United States proved too costly, they settled on a clinic in Mumbai that was well known for providing surrogacy services to gay couples from around the world.

The next step in the process—selecting an egg donor—was a difficult task for Aaron and Ben. The couple considered Indian egg donation but had issues with the lack of available medical data:

> We found that India doesn't have a population registry, so we didn't want to do the egg donation here because you couldn't get a medical history. When you do egg donation in the States or another place, you get like three generations of medical data of the donor and her family and stuff like that, which you couldn't do here. So we started by finding egg donations in other places, and we actually ended up having an egg donor in Romania, to which we sent sperm, and the eggs were fertilized and frozen in Romania, then shipped to India.

While Aaron and Ben emphasized the importance of the availability of a medical history in selecting an egg donor, they simultaneously assumed that genetic influences on physical and psychological characteristics were straightforward and deterministic, reflecting a common view perpetuated by donor agencies (Daniels and Heidt-Forsythe 2012; Thompson 2009). In pursuit of an egg provider with a robust medical history file, Aaron and Ben commissioned multiple IVF attempts with frozen embryos. Interestingly, however, the couple's search took them to countries in which the ideal "three generations of medical data" was not always obtainable; instead, the availability of even a minimal medical history justified the around-the-world search for suitable eggs. They sought parenthood through a Romanian egg donor agency and then one based in the United States, both of which involved frozen embryos that didn't take. Ultimately they arranged for a young, white South African egg donor to fly to Mumbai for egg retrieval and the transfer of the fresh embryo to an Indian surrogate. Several weeks prior to my first meeting with Aaron and Ben, their surrogate, Sarita, gave birth via cesarean section to twin girls, Tara and Noelle.

Ben's mother, Shari, had accompanied Aaron and Ben to India, and I spoke with all three of them about Tara and Noelle's relationship with both the egg donor and Sarita, their surrogate. This was a topic of great concern for Aaron, who had been concerned from the beginning about the ethical and moral issues related to surrogacy. At our very first meeting, he reported that he and Ben wanted to do everything they could to "minimize the possibility of the surrogate mother feeling that she was used. And if possible, even to let her finish the process with her feeling that she has done something noble and that she can be proud of herself." Indeed, Aaron had met with Sarita prior to the twins' birth, and he described the meeting this way: "My emphasis was to try and show her my gratitude and to make sure that she feels that I don't take advantage, and that I don't take this as part of a business transaction." During his stay in Mumbai, Aaron had hoped that he might be able to arrange another meeting with Sarita and her family, in part to get to know her better but also to reassure himself that Sarita was at peace with the experience of surrogacy.

Shari, on the other hand, did not share Aaron's concern and it was clear the two had already debated this issue. When I asked whether he had been able to meet with Sarita yet, Aaron replied:

> No . . . I haven't, I still want to do it . . . but we have different thoughts about it within the family. I think it should be done. But Shari thinks that our desire to keep up with Sarita or maintain contact with her is like some sort of avoidance, like we are avoiding the "real" mother, the genetic mother. Shari thinks that the genetic donor is probably the person that the girls will be more interested in.

I asked Aaron what he thought about the egg donor's relationship to his children. Aaron said:

Well, first of all, I think her involvement is much shorter. She comes from a much closer background to us, she's Western . . . and she went through a short process. I'm less worried about her well-being in a way. I think her experience was less intensive. I think if the girls decide they want to go after her, I'm less worried about it. . . . They will probably be able to track her down and she will probably be just a regular person. . . . I'm not afraid of what they will think regarding us and our relationship with the donor. All that is different from what I'm thinking about Sarita. I think that if they find Sarita, as a low-middle class lady in India, it will be a culture shock. Somehow I think the bond of carrying a baby for nine months is more important than a medical procedure where you have eggs extracted. I think that there is a better chance that Sarita will be contemplating what happened with the two babies, than the donor.

Throughout the course of our interviews, Aaron returned to this contrast between the white woman who contributed her eggs and Sarita, who contributed the work of gestation, labor, and delivery. He also said that he couldn't do anything for the egg donor whereas he viewed Sarita as a poor woman in India who could benefit from his goodwill: "There are things I can do. I can keep in touch with her. I can take care of her and see if there's anything I can do to help her in the future." Aaron's feeling of compulsion to act as benefactor to Sarita reveals his consciousness of the unequal relationship inherent in his surrogacy experience and the broader stratification of reproduction at work.

Aaron's narrative also reflects the script of rescue prevalent among commissioning parents pursuing surrogacy in India. While Shari argued that the genetic material provided by the egg donor signals "real" motherhood, Aaron wanted their surrogate to feel "noble," thus making her worthy of saving. Aaron consistently avoided the language of commodification, reiterating that his relationship with Sarita was more than a "business transaction." For Aaron, then, the kinship between Sarita and his twin girls was a complicated one. Aaron viewed the labor of gestation and delivery as stronger and more enduring than the genetic connection between the egg donor and the girls, even though his daughters' relationship with their surrogate mother traversed class, race, and national divides. Yet feeling deeply conflicted about the hierarchies of nationality and class that permeated this relationship, Aaron sought to mitigate these tensions by relying on narratives of rescue. In doing so, however, Aaron depended on constructions of Sarita as fundamentally Other from himself, his children, and even the egg donor, whom he viewed as "just a regular person." Sarita, in contrast, was viewed as essentially different, "a low-middle class lady in India" who signified Otherness through her race, culture, and nationality.

Patricia, a forty-four-year-old mother of a son born through surrogacy in India, also referred to the nobility of surrogacy work. Patricia and her husband, Jonas, a white married couple from the United States, suffered problems with infertility and pursued surrogacy in India with an Indian egg donor, primarily for reasons of cost. While she was very focused on the selection of the egg donor, Patricia said that with regard to the surrogate, "I just let the doctors pick who they thought would be a good candidate. I didn't really focus on that selection as much because I didn't really think it was that important; I just assumed that through their screening process they'd identify anyone who was not fit for pregnancy." In contrast to other commissioning parents that revered the bond between the surrogate and fetus, Patricia's primary concern was with physical fitness for pregnancy. After meeting the surrogate, she realized, however, that she did not share their doctor's judgment of fitness for pregnancy:

> The thing that most struck us about her was how tiny she was. The paperwork said that she was about 5'1" and when we met her in person—I'm 5'1" and I towered over her, so she was about 4'9", maybe. I think the day before she gave birth she weighed 110 pounds, so when we met before she was pregnant she was probably about 85 pounds. We never would have picked her if we had known how small she was.

Here, Patricia's discussion of the surrogate's "fitness" and size were euphemistic terms for race. In a tone of disbelief, Patricia remarked on the small stature of the surrogate. Yet even though the surrogate had previously given birth to her own healthy children, Patricia implicitly suggested that she was too small to give birth to her (white) child. The difference in size substituted a discussion of racial difference; indeed, ethnographic accounts have revealed how American couples voice concerns over Indian women's small physical size, believing that she would not be able to carry a healthy pregnancy to term (Rudrappa 2014). The surrogate's "fitness" notwithstanding, everything turned out fine, as Patricia explained, and their son was born healthy, if several weeks premature.

When I asked about her relationship with the surrogate, Patricia replied:

> We met her when we signed the initial contract. She was a very, very shy woman. The doctors that we were working with offered to intermediate, but it was very awkward. We didn't really know what to say to her or how to talk to her. Through the paperwork we learned that she had been married at about fourteen and had her first baby around that age and a second baby still in her teens. We had one phone call with her during the pregnancy, and again, because the doctors were intermediating, she was very shy and deferential to them. So we really didn't have a direct connection with her.

Patricia's communication with her surrogate mirrored the experience of many couples I interviewed, who noted the awkwardness that permeated their interactions. While parents rely on doctors and clinic staff to mediate conversations with surrogates, who rarely speak any English, they acknowledge the difficulty of nurturing any kind of "direct connection," despite their desire for one. Moreover, Patricia leaned on the mythical stereotype of the submissive, deferential Asian woman in the absence of any intimate connection or knowledge of their surrogate as an individual.

Within this context, the rescue script came to the fore. Patricia went on to explain a subsequent meeting with the surrogate's family:

> We had one other interesting interaction with regard to the surrogate: when we came back we brought over some things for her children. Just a few backpacks filled with school and art supplies, nothing major. But I gave it to her husband because she was already being admitted to the hospital. And he fell to the floor and kissed my feet! And that was just such a strange moment for me. We were already very emotional, but I think that really gave us an insight into what impact this was having on their family, this money she was earning and the opportunity she was earning. In the

one photo we got of her when she was pregnant, she looked like she had so much pride in what she was doing. It made us feel good, that she was doing something that she could do very easily and yet it was making an impact on her and her family. I guess we were worried that people might judge us for being exploitative or somehow taking advantage of people who were too poor to be making their own decisions, but we didn't feel that way. We felt like everyone was making out in this situation.

Like Aaron, Patricia projected an idea of nobility and pride onto her surrogate. In foregrounding the surrogate's "pride" in what she could do for her family, Patricia romanticized the surrogate's role. She also highlighted Indian culture as exotic, strange, and essentially different— exclaiming how "strange" it was for her when her surrogate's husband kissed her feet—in order to normalize this means of family formation. At the same time, Patricia deemphasized the surrogate's position as a mother to her own child conceived through ART, as she expressed deeper concern about the selection of an egg donor.

Patricia also divulged her perception of the risks involved in being a surrogate; she seriously downplayed the risks and labor involved in gestation and childbirth, describing pregnancy as something that could be done "very easily." While Patricia's comments reflect the views implicit in the ICMR's Draft Bill that diminish the risks and labor associated with surrogacy, surrogates' experiences indicate otherwise, and the labor involved in surrogacy is by no means easy. Yet emphasizing notions of rescue and nobility shifts the focus onto the surrogate as an object to be saved and conceals the physical labor, pain, and risks that she endures.

"It's a Business Transaction": Other Forms of Reciprocity

While narratives of rescue dominated many conversations, not all the parents in this study relied on rescue scripts in their narratives about family making through surrogacy. Rather than conceal the commodifying aspects of surrogacy through claims of humanitarianism, about a dozen intended parents I interviewed embraced the transactional nature of commercial surrogacy. Some intended parents, as I will explain, began their surrogacy journeys with a strong desire to develop close bonds with their surrogate but began to think of surrogacy as a straightforward business transaction under the stress of needing to make multiple IVF attempts. Heterosexual married women who had medical histories of infertility and underwent multiple surrogacy attempts in India seemed to be the most likely to undergo this change, although four gay male respondents also described surrogacy in transactional terms.

Jan, for example, saw her views of surrogacy shift over time, particularly as she encountered conflicts with her doctor over the management of her first surrogate pregnancy in Mumbai. In the beginning, she says, "I was really into the touchy feely thing, 'Let's all be extended family, let's have belly shots, let's give presents.'" She had commissioned the pregnancy through a clinic that tried to foster relationships between intended parents and surrogates through Skype, phone calls, and shared photographs of the pregnant woman's growing belly; the doctors in this practice supported parents' wishes to give gifts to surrogates during the pregnancy. Gift giving seemed to represent a kind of reciprocity for the reproductive labor. Yet Jan later came to feel that gift giving "puts so much stress, not just on the surrogates, but their families because they don't give presents back." She explained,

> We think about the surrogates every day and we wish we could do more. But it's actually an intrusion on them to receive these crap gifts that we send. I know somebody gave a sterling silver necklace to his surrogate after the baby was born, and that's an insult in India! Like, 18 carat is an insult; they're all 22 carat gold. So it's just not understanding the customs, and the fact is that I know the majority of us, if not everybody, will want to [give gifts], but we have to wait [until after the child is born].

Gift giving across cultural boundaries was a topic of heated debate among intended parents. I observed that intended parents consulted each other over appropriate gifts, and doctors began to realize that gift giving resulted in competition and jealousy among surrogates. When Jan decided to try a different clinic, she explained that her new doctor did not encourage gift giving during pregnancy:

> [The doctor] says, no, give them [presents] later. And we will gift our surrogate later. We've met our surrogate, we've got photos of her, I constantly inquire about her, I constantly think about her. I would love to

send her presents, but I know that once the baby is delivered, *she will be gifted very handsomely by us* [emphasis added]. Which we don't have to do; we want to do that. But it's the rules to do it this way and I agree with her. After being through it before, and you see on some of the blogs, "Oh, we're extended family . . ." I know now that's bullshit, that's absolute crap! They're not. You get your baby, you give them a bonus, you go home, you've got your baby. The thing is, it doesn't mean we don't think about our surrogate. It doesn't mean we're not going to send them presents.

Disillusioned with efforts at making kinship with surrogates, Jan came to view surrogacy as a purely transactional relationship, much like one between an employer and a worker who receives a "bonus" upon completion of her job. Though she did not believe in gift giving during pregnancy, she felt strongly that parents should give gifts after the child was born. "Our surrogate's got a child and I know that she's going to spend a lot of the compensation on educating that child. We're actually going to pay for that child's education so she doesn't have to use her compensation. And that's going to be our gift to her." Here, the gift becomes a reciprocal act not for the surrogate's labor, which takes place throughout the pregnancy, but for the end product, the child.

Similarly, Lucy, a thirty-six-year-old Australian woman pursuing surrogacy in Delhi, changed her views of surrogacy over a period of several months. Unlike most intended parents in this study, Lucy already had two daughters, aged eleven and eight. Lucy and her husband always imagined they would have four children, yet she endured difficult pregnancies with both her children. After postpartum hemorrhaging following the birth of her second child, Lucy had to have a hysterectomy. For years, Lucy said, she and her husband "mourned not having another child." Upon learning about surrogacy in India, Lucy saw an opportunity to achieve her dream of having more children.

Although Lucy did not have a uterus, her ovaries functioned normally, and she and her husband arranged their first trip to India with plans for Lucy to undergo egg retrieval in Delhi. Embryos created with Lucy's eggs and her husband's sperm were transferred to the surrogate, and on the first attempt their surrogate became pregnant. But when the surrogate later miscarried, Lucy was heartbroken. The couple quickly regrouped, however, and planned a second trip to India. As she was preparing to undergo a second egg retrieval and surrogacy attempt in India, I asked Lucy about her perspective on the surrogacy process and her relationship with the surrogate. She replied:

> When I met my first surrogate who was pregnant, I loved her. I thought she was beautiful and just wonderful. But I've changed my opinion on how I want to know them now. At first, I wanted to know them and everything about them and talk to them. But I think after our miscarriage, I'm probably changing to, "Look, this is a business deal." I can't get attached to them; I want the best surrogate I can get. And I probably want to put a little more business relationship into it than last time. I think that I don't want to get too attached. And I was asked [by the doctor] if I want to use the same surrogate again, and I don't. I want to broaden my chances of trying something else, and I probably don't need to meet them this time.

Like Jan, the changes in Lucy's views were associated with early disappointments and failed attempts at surrogacy. With the low rates of success in surrogacy, intended parents like Jan and Lucy often become increasingly businesslike in their approach as they undergo multiple surrogacy attempts. As a result, Lucy believed that it was unnecessary to meet, learn about, or develop a relationship with the woman who would carry her potential child. Instead, she became occupied with the business aspects of surrogacy; in Lucy's case, her main concern was with finding the "best surrogate she could get." Here, Lucy was not concerned with finding a woman she can "rescue." Rather, her goal was to find the woman whose reproductive body would fulfill the job she is being hired to do: gestate and give birth to a healthy child for Lucy and her husband.

Yet Lucy's idea of the suitable reproductive body rested on specific racial constructions of India and Indian people.

> The people here are absolutely beautiful. They are just an amazing race; so kind. And one of the biggest things I can tell you that stays in my mind is that they dress so well and look after themselves so well—with nothing! That doesn't compare to what we have. And they look so beautiful, everyone's so clean! And the driving, I must admit, there's no lanes, no

indicators, there's just honking. I don't think I was quite prepared. It's like Bangkok or Bali. But I have no qualms or questions about doing surrogacy in India. It was just wonderful.

Like other intended parents I interviewed, Lucy held deeply romanticized and exoticized views of India. She explicitly referred to Indians as an "amazing race," expressing a certain narrative about India as exotic and filled with beauty. Moreover, through an Orientalist gaze, Lucy constructed Indians explicitly in opposition to Westerners, shocked that they could "look so beautiful" despite their poverty. Yet she simultaneously portrayed India as chaotic and disordered, clearly marking India as Other to her familiar suburban Australia, and similar to other Third World cities like Bangkok or Bali. In doing so, as Laura Harrison suggests, Lucy "reifies racial difference through euphemistic devices that posit India as the excessive, fertile maternal body in contrast to the deserving, but barren Western woman" (2014, 151). This trope established the child's belonging with her or her white parents.

Karen, a forty-one-year-old Australian mother of twin boys born via surrogacy, echoed Jan's and Lucy's sentiments about the transactional character of surrogacy. More than a decade ago and prior to meeting her husband, Karen was diagnosed with cervical cancer. As part of her treatment, Karen underwent a hysterectomy. Yet, Karen explained, "I knew I had a need to nurture," and she and her husband explored international adoption before realizing that "it just seemed impossible" due to the low rates of domestic adoption in Australia and the long waiting periods for international adoption.

Then Karen learned about surrogacy, and immediately went to an IVF clinic to find out whether her ovaries still functioned. She was thrilled to learn that her own eggs were still viable. At the same time, once Karen started to explore surrogacy options, she knew that she would need to go abroad. While altruistic surrogacy is permitted in Australia, commercial surrogacy is not, and Karen felt strongly about compensating the surrogate: "If I was going to be trusting someone, another woman, to carry a baby for me, I needed certainty that she was going to hand it over. So we wanted to pay a surrogate for that reason. I want to compensate her, I want it to be a commercial relationship, and I want that baby." Eventually, Karen and her husband decided to work with a clinic in Mumbai, and after one negative result and one miscarriage, Karen's surrogate became pregnant with twins on their third try.

Unlike most of my respondents who deemphasized the transactional nature of surrogacy, Karen entered into the arrangement with this emphasis. Yet Karen's surrogacy experience, which occurred in the year prior to our interview, was far from uncomplicated. Once she learned that her surrogate, Mona, was carrying twins, Karen was overjoyed. Mona and her husband, however, had major concerns regarding the risks associated with multifetal pregnancy. Moreover, they knew that surrogates who gestated twins often received higher payments, and Mona's husband wanted to ensure they would receive the highest payment to which they were entitled; he argued that they should receive double the amount originally cited in the contract. Karen and her husband had planned to travel to India to see the first heartbeat scan of the fetus (at around eight weeks' gestation), and on the day of the scan Karen learned that Mona and her husband wanted to do a "selective reduction" procedure to terminate one of the embryos. As Karen explained, "We were told that if we didn't approve the selective reduction, the surrogate would disappear and they would terminate the entire pregnancy." Karen turned to the doctors at their surrogacy agency for help in mediating the conflict and managing the pregnancy. Everything they did, as Karen described, "was an effort to buy time, so that they'd get to the stage where [Mona and her husband] couldn't terminate the pregnancy." For the majority of the pregnancy, she says, "We were faced with the fact that if we didn't pay, [the surrogate's husband] was going to take her back to his village and just terminate the pregnancy or leave the babies on the side of the road to die. We had no idea what was going to happen."

Yet though Karen agreed to pay for Mona's child's primary school education, something she had planned to do anyway, Karen learned that Mona and her husband never received this information. Karen would later become highly critical of the ways in which the doctors mismanaged the pregnancy and bungled communications. She attributed many of these problems to "culture," understood as indicators of difference that are both unchangeable and difficult to negotiate. Here, culture "can be appreciated as 'data about individual racial thoughts and fantasies' insofar as culture and race have begun to proceed to the same effect"

(Bridges 2011, 136). Karen's notion of culture-as-race served to Other not only Indian surrogates but also the doctors who stood in for the nation of India.

With only Karen's version of the story available to me, it is difficult to know exactly what Mona and her husband were thinking or to estimate the seriousness of their threats to end the pregnancy. Nonetheless, Karen came to believe that she and her husband were being "held hostage for the entire pregnancy." As she explained:

> I don't know how, but my surrogate's husband was in charge of my preg-
> nancy. So my husband went over at 32 weeks because we knew that the
> twins would be viable and that was the point that Mona could deliver
> them. He went with her to an obstetrics appointment at the hospital and
> managed to get the surrogate admitted. And she was threatened that if
> she left the hospital she'd be arrested for kidnapping. I got there a week
> later and we tried to work out what was going on.

Eventually, Karen, her husband, and the doctors made plans to deliver the twins via cesarean section at thirty-four weeks' gestation, even though the surgery was not medically indicated. Evidently, Karen and her husband viewed Mona—construed here as a potential kidnapper of children—as a greater threat to their children than the health risks of premature delivery via cesarean section.

Yet when Karen and her husband arrived at the hospital on the day of the scheduled birth, they learned that Mona had refused to sign the consent form for surgery. According to Karen, the doctor at the surrogacy agency explained to Mona that she would not be receiving any extra payments, despite the fact that Karen insisted she had agreed to offer more money. Under these circumstances, the hospital did not want to "get involved" and refused to proceed with the surgery. The hospital's fear, Karen explained, was that without Mona's signature on the consent form, Mona could potentially claim that the children were taken from her against her will, thus challenging one of the core claims of Indian surrogacy proponents: that surrogates always and willingly hand over the babies to their rightful parents. Karen went on to describe a scene that sounded chaotic, as Karen, her husband, and Mona and her husband were ordered to leave the hospital, while their doctors scrambled to find an alternative hospital in which Mona could give birth. While the clinic's lawyers suggested "calling their bluff" and allowing Mona and her husband to leave the hospital, Karen refused to let them "disappear" and insisted, "These children are being delivered now." Eventually, the twins were born in a local clinic and transferred to a nearby NICU, where one newborn would spend one week, and the other, three.

However, despite all the tension, confusion, and uncertainty Karen experienced throughout the surrogacy process, she continued to describe surrogacy in India as "viable." But she was clear how she believed commissioning parents should proceed:

> I think you have to go into it as a business transaction. You are not going to make friends with your surrogate. I actually advise people to not even meet your surrogate. Don't meet her; meet her after birth. It's not going to be like if we had a surrogate in America that we could talk to, Skype, email, any of that. For example, we were trying to send some extra money to our surrogate at some point, and no one in her entire family had photographic ID to go pick up a Western Union money transfer. They likely have a mobile phone but she doesn't speak English. She wouldn't know how to turn a computer on. And I'm not trying to be rude here; but we're employing her. It's as simple as that. It's a business transaction. She's doing her job; she gets paid for it. Thank you very much; you'll always be dear to my heart, end of story.

Karen's experience led her to believe that the ideal conditions for surrogacy were those that articulated a strictly transactional relationship. She cautioned that prospective parents should have no illusions about the relationship they would have with the surrogate; surrogates and clients should not become friends, nor should they meet in person prior to the birth. Yet Karen also signaled the wide power disparity between Indian surrogates and women like herself from more prosperous nations. With a U.S. surrogate, she argued, one could Skype, email, and hold meaningful conversations. Indian surrogates, on the other hand, might not even "know how to turn a computer on." They are constructed as naïve and ignorant, the opposite of modern, and their supposed ignorance is often revealing of their attribution as a racialized and classed Other. Such constructions reveal how race operates implicitly in the context of transnational surrogacy; assumptions about Third World difference and what Banerjee calls "First World privilege" (2014, 122) illustrate how a surrogate's location in a developing country heavily influence white, Western fertility travelers' perceptions of her. Racial difference and racial hierarchies are implied, particularly across the First World/Third World divide: "As a result, such stereotypes as the 'poor Third World woman of color,' oppressed within her own society, continue to be perpetuated within a neocolonial space" (Banerjee 2010, 118).

Yet even as Karen viewed Indian surrogates as uneducated, she simultaneously considered Mona and her husband to be incredibly shrewd. The mythology of the duplicitous surrogate relies on the coexistence of these two characteristics, ignorance and duplicity, within the surrogate patient. But this mythology is contradictory; if surrogates were as ignorant as doctors and commissioning parents believe them to be, they would lack the intelligence to manipulate and blackmail commissioning parents. Nonetheless, Indian surrogates embody this paradox, and the intersection of these contradictions is visible in mainstream and popular representations of surrogates. In their examination of the public inquiry that preceded the passing of the Surrogacy Bill (2010) in New South Wales, Australia, Riggs and Due (2012) illustrate how the construction of women and motherhood devalued women who act as surrogates while also asserting their status as the child's "proper" mother. In other words, women who act as surrogates are simultaneously referred to as mothers and treated as already being failed mothers for carrying and giving away a child. Similarly, Teman (2008) has found that the majority of the psychosocial literature that examines the surrogate's experience portrays her as economically desperate, in need of psychological reparation, or possessing abnormal personality characteristics. These representations ultimately frame the surrogate as deviant, deceitful, and incapable of rationally choosing and negotiating surrogacy arrangements.

Karen's language concurrently evokes the ways in which an employer might speak about a poor, uneducated worker. Though Jan, Lucy, and Karen rejected the rescue narrative and embraced a business framework for narrating their surrogacy journey, they embraced hierarchy through an employer-worker script. Jan, Lucy, and Karen still controlled the terms of the transaction. In this case, the "job" that surrogates take up is not defined by the labor that goes into pregnancy and childbirth, but by the end product of this labor, a healthy child. By devaluing the surrogate's labor and focusing on the product of the transaction, such narratives place the surrogate in a precarious position should anything go awry during the pregnancy.

In her work on adoption in the United States, Christine Gailey (2010, 117) highlights the processual nature of kinship through what she calls substantiation:

> *Substantiation* is what I call the process through which people enter and are embraced in a web of sharing, obligation, reciprocal claiming, and emotional and material support that is considered the most sustaining kind of kinship or family. It is a process of naming, asserting connection, and pooling material and non-material resources that, depending on its intensity, can carve out what Richard Lee terms a "safety net" for participants, the closest degree of kinship, regardless of state definitions of "family" (see Lee 1992).

Building on Gailey's notion of substantiation, I suggest that in the context of transnational surrogacy, kinship is a complex chain of events, something located in everyday practices and experiences and informed by ideologies of race. As I have shown, many parents interviewed held contradictory views of kinship that simultaneously destabilized and reinforced dominant ideologies of kinship that emphasize ties based on blood. I found that in general, certain groups of parents held similar views of kinship, though these often overlapped. For instance, those who explicitly mentioned a desire to "pass on" their lineage—to have a genetically related child—tended to be heterosexual individuals who did not use egg donation (though a few gay male parents also fell into this category). On the other hand, those who deemphasized the importance of genetic relationships tended to be using egg donation and were equally balanced between gay and straight couples. There were still others, both gay and straight, who were ambivalent about the role of genetics.

These views of kinship overlapped with commissioning parents' racial imaginaries that alternately revolve around narratives of rescue and remuneration. In general, individuals who deemphasized biogenetic kinship tended to embrace rescue narratives. Those who sought to reinforce the importance of biogenetic kinship, on the other hand, embraced a more transactional view of surrogacy that emphasized surrogates' remuneration. In both cases, commissioning parents embraced racial ideologies that Othered Indian surrogates, reinforced Orientalist constructions of India and Indian women, and reified racial hierarchies implied in First World/Third World divides. I contend that the ways in which ideas of kinship and parenthood intersect with notions of rescue and narratives of transaction ultimately maintain and reinforce global structures of stratification.

Taking up Charis Thompson's (2001) claim that "biological" kinship may be configured in multiple ways, I suggest that there is no "unique template" for kinship within the context of transnational surrogacy. Indeed, as I will discuss further in chapter 3, the commodification of race in the context of gamete donation both challenges and reconfigures understandings of biological, genetic, and adoptive kinship in unexpected ways.

3

Egg Donation and Exotic Beauty

The womb is like an oven. It merely bakes the cake. Whether
you insert a chocolate or strawberry cake is for you to decide.
—Fertility doctor, quoted in Jaisinghani, *Maid-to-Order
Surrogate Mums*

When Jan Marks booked her first trip to India to begin the surrogacy
process in December 2008, she arranged for a young white woman
to travel to India for the purposes of egg donation. At the time, Jan
explained, "I really wanted a child that looked like me: tall, blond,
blue-eyed, that kind of thing. . . . I was really concerned—because I've
never had a baby before—that I wouldn't love a baby as much if it didn't
look like me." Jan believed that her unusual path to parenthood would
require the assistance of an Indian surrogate mother and a young, white
egg donor. Thus she chose to work with a surrogacy agency in Mumbai
that had connections with a South African egg donor agency tasked with
coordinating the recruitment of primarily white women willing to travel
as egg donors.

Yet after several surrogacy attempts ended in miscarriage, Jan had a
change of heart regarding the particular phenotypic characteristics she
desired in her child. Worried about their shrinking budget, the couple
decided to continue pursuing parenthood through gestational surrogacy, but with an Indian egg donor whose fees would be significantly
lower than those of the South African donor.[1] When I asked her about
this change, Jan replied, "When I'd flown in this South African donor
and it didn't work, part of the grief was, 'Oh my god, I'm never going
to have a blond, blue-eyed child now!'" But she went on to elaborate
that she felt "quite proud" of her decision to use an Indian egg donor.
While Jan described herself as "quite fair," she explained that despite her
Polish-Scottish heritage, most of her family has darker, olive-toned skin:
"A dark child is actually going to fit in well with the family! And hon-

estly, she [the egg donor] is the spitting image of my sister when she was younger. . . . So I carry that donor's photo around with me in my wallet, because I'm just—I'm going to get emotional—but I'm just so grateful." Interestingly, as Jan navigated the disappointment of not being able to have a child that resembled her physically, she took comfort in the fact that her Indian egg donor resembled her sister and that the child would fit in with her darker-skinned extended family.

This chapter explores the ways in which commissioning parents pursuing surrogacy in India negotiate the process of third-party egg donation. As the epigraph suggests, Indian medical doctors draw attention to the marketlike aspects of gestational surrogacy and egg donation, comparing the process of creating a life (with specified phenotypic or skin color characteristics) to the simple consumer choice of whether to select a "chocolate or strawberry cake." I examine the ways in which intended parents and doctors navigate such choices through the practice of transnational egg donation. In particular, I analyze the ways in which commissioning parents construct relations with the egg provider—the genetic parent of the child—as well as with the child conceived through egg donation, IVF, and gestational surrogacy. I also explore the means through which doctors organize practices of transnational and local egg donation. While egg donors undoubtedly play a central role in this process as the providers of genetic material, in what follows I focus primarily on the perspectives of doctors and commissioning parents, as I am interested in how these actors, the organizers and consumers of assisted reproduction, deploy notions of race, nationality, and skin color in the context of egg donation. By examining doctors' and commissioning parents' narratives, I illustrate the heterogeneity of approaches to egg donation in the context of neoliberal global forces that place the onus on egg purchasers to "choose" the genetic material of future children.

The connections between surrogacy, commerce, and choice are worth elaborating briefly. ART use, including IVF, egg donation, and gestational surrogacy, are typically represented simply as infertility treatment. Yet this framing focuses the gaze on the medical aspects of assisted reproduction. These treatments, however, occur within a much larger, wide-ranging set of activities that are commercial in nature and constitute the basis of the fertility industry—an industry that

has expanded across national borders to promote the growth of reproductive tourism around the globe. Within this global fertility market,
racial identity figures prominently, as ART consumers who seek third-
party gametes often have particular racial preferences.[2] Many, for instance, seek gametes from donors of similar racial background, while
others pursue gametes from distinct backgrounds, as in the case of a
white German couple who selected an Indian egg donor because they
hoped the resulting child might reflect their interest in Buddhism (even
though it was unlikely that the Indian donor was actually Buddhist)
(Thompson 2009). Such racial preferences influence demand in the international market, making race a commodity to be selected, acquired,
and purchased. However, in the context of assisted reproduction, the
ability to "choose" race naturalizes other genetic preferences, making
them seem "both natural and acceptable, thus clouding what might
otherwise seem to be obvious eugenic preferences" (Ikemoto 2009,
308). In other words, by validating race as a consumable good, private
commerce clears the way for condoning the commodification of many
other traits, reinforcing notions of genetic essentialism, veiling eugenic
preferences, and viewing difference through a "prism of heritability"
(Browner and Press 1995, 307).

As Western parents pursue surrogacy and egg donation in India,
they make reproductive decisions within a framework of transnational
inequalities along national, racial/ethnic, and class lines. I found that
for many parents, this process is most intense and intimate within the
context of egg donation. Their narratives reveal the diversity of ways in
which they address issues of phenotype, genetics, and kinship. Scholars
have suggested that the fertility industry serves to reproduce the hegemonic white patriarchal family, arguing that white Western couples
will avoid using eggs from a different racial background (Cooper and
Waldby 2014; Banerjee 2014; Quiroga 2007). As Banerjee states, "Although white Western couples are ready to avail themselves of the services of the Indian surrogates, they predominantly refrain from using
eggs and sperm from a different racial group" (2014, 123). Yet in contrast
to dominant assumptions that intended parents primarily seek donors
who match their own phenotypic or ethnic backgrounds, I found that
of the 19 mostly white couples/individuals who used donor eggs in their
surrogacy process, 11 commissioning couples who identified as white

sought Indian egg donors with darker skin tones; three couples who identified as mixed did as well. I suggest that while such actions appear to subvert dominant hierarchies that privilege white skin, revealing potential spaces of resistance to racialized preconceptions about kinship, they in fact rely on essentialized notions of race and beauty and reflect new articulations of biological race. Here, I argue that Indian/Asian racial Otherness emerges as a desirable commodity whose value is enhanced precisely as a result of its consumption at the global level. In other words, racialized gametes offer the consumer a product linked to place, history, and difference; thus, it becomes part of a family's kinship narrative, a story of people and places that in turn marks the child as authentically "Indian."

Defining Race and Skin Color: Identity and Notions of Essentialism

Jan's story of her path to transnational surrogacy and egg donation raises several questions. How do commissioning parents navigate the process of selecting an egg provider, specifically for the purposes of conception via IVF and gestational surrogacy? What factors might prompt a Western couple pursuing surrogacy in India to select a white egg provider from another country? Alternatively, why might a couple select a darker-skinned Indian egg provider? How do Indian doctors convey the various options available to clients in terms of race, skin color, or ethnicity? These questions point to broader issues about the intersections between race, kinship, and assisted reproduction: what do these stories tell us about how intended parents understand the relationship between race, nationality, genetics, and kinship? What do these narratives reveal about the broader stratification of reproduction?

In addressing these questions, it is important to first clarify how commissioning parents and Indian doctors understand notions of race, skin color, nationality, and ethnicity. In the context of transnational surrogacy, I encountered a range of systems of racial and skin color classification among non-Indian commissioning parents and Indian doctors and surrogates. These actors, hailing from different nations, often expressed different understandings of race, skin color, nationality, and ethnicity which at times intersected and overlapped in the process of transnational reproduction. Often actors conflated notions of race, skin color, nationality, and ethnicity.

Foreign commissioning parents traveling to India, for instance, tend to rely on racial categories that reflect Western notions of race based on phenotype. Parents of children conceived with Indian donor eggs and the intended father's sperm often described their children as "biracial" or "mixed-race," meaning they were part Indian and part white, with the understanding that Indians were racially classified as "Asian" as per U.S. census categories. Commissioning parents often conflated this notion of race with ideas of nationality and culture in ways I will discuss further in this chapter. Some intended parents, for example, believing that eggs from an Indian woman would make their child "part Indian" through the conferral of certain skin color and other physical characteristics, simultaneously felt a responsibility to teach their children about their "Indian heritage." These parents spoke of educating their children about Indian foods, culture, and religious rituals. Further complicating this picture is the belief of still other parents that it was not genetics, but gestation, that bestowed on children some degree of "Indian" heritage and identity (Deomampo 2013).

In India too the category of race is a complex issue. During British colonial rule in India, various attempts were made to classify the Indian population according to a racial typology, reflecting the predominant racial theories popular in nineteenth-century Europe. Following India's independence from British rule, the 1951 Census of India abolished racial classifications, and today the national census does not recognize any racial groups in India. Yet scholars have argued that "race lives through the category of caste as a form of racial Indianization" (Das 2014, 278). Caste is classified into Forward Caste (Brahmins and other propertied castes), Scheduled Caste (SC) and Scheduled Tribe (ST), and Other Backward Classes (OBCs) comprised of "socially and educationally backward classes" (Deshpande 2005, 3). While the SC category encompasses Dalits and other historically disadvantaged caste groups, ST consists of geographically isolated communities.

However, the relationship between caste and race is controversial in India. In 2001, Dalit activists successfully campaigned to include caste discrimination on the agenda of the World Conference against Racism, Racial Discrimination and Xenophobia in Durban. Various constituents, including the Indian government and Indian sociologists, strongly opposed these efforts, denying any association between caste and race. Several scholars have strongly objected to arguments that caste is equal to race, arguing that historical attempts to categorize Indians into racial groups are inaccurate. Indeed, Beteille (2001) points out that attempts to distinguish between Aryan and Dravidian races during colonial times "were linguistic or regional categories in disguise and not racial categories at all." He further argues that "the metaphor of race is a dangerous weapon whether it is used for asserting white supremacy or for making demands on behalf of disadvantaged groups" (Beteille 2001), and thus caste discrimination cannot be treated as a form of racial discrimination. Yet as Natrajan and Greenough contend, "it is not that caste is race, but that racism and casteism have comparable effects; they are both processes of oppression that depend on the 'naturalization' of race and caste" (cited in Baber 2010, 246).

Thus caste, like race, assumes its power through the specific contexts in which it is embedded. Indeed, just as racial categories are essentialized as immutable and inheritable, caste groups too are essentialized and racialized through "quasi-biological overtones, such as fair, upper-caste Brahmins and dark, lower-caste non-Brahmins" (Das 2014, 271). Although individuals of fair and dark skin tone can be found at all levels of caste and class in India, in general dark skin is linked with lower castes while fair-skinned individuals enjoy greater wealth and social status.

In the context of egg donation, then, skin color, not race, is perhaps the most salient organizing feature. By skin color, I refer to subjective understandings of skin color or tone which span different terminologies, depending on the context. Many South Asian languages, for example, have terms to refer to different shades of skin tone. In Hindi, *gora/gori* refers to fair or light-skinned individuals, *saanwala* refers to wheatish brown skin, and *kala/kali* means black, or dark skin. In Punjabi, a person's fair complexion is compared to the color of milk (*dudh waken*) or to the color of the moon; a dark person's complexion, on the other hand, is likened to that of a crow or the back of an iron skillet (Vaid 2009, 148). In one Mumbai IVF clinic, skin color is described on an egg donor profile form along a spectrum of shades, including dark, dark wheatish, wheatish (light brown), light wheatish, fair, and very fair.

Interestingly, however, with the increase in global consumers of ARTs traveling to India, Indian doctors are increasingly adopting the language of race in their interactions with foreign clients. Indeed, elites in China and Japan historically have drawn inspiration from scientific racism, taking up Western notions of race in order to buttress indigenous discourses of difference and in some instances, stratify internal and external populations (Dikötter 1997; Weiner 1997). This adds yet another layer of complexity to understandings of race in the Indian context, as Indian doctors, who rely on categories of caste and religion in their own social contexts, utilize Western categories of race in the global spheres of transnational reproduction.

These categories—of race, nationality, skin color, and ethnicity—and the varied ways in which actors understand, conflate, and define them, hold critical implications for notions of identity and essentialism in the context of reproductive technology. Anthropologists have long examined the ways in which "identity" is an unstable object of inquiry. Rather than being immutable, identity is not considered to be a fixed essence, and scholars have explored how individuals craft their identities through social performances. However, with the increasing availability of and reliance on reproductive and genetic technologies, essentialist identities have grown ever more powerful. New genetic knowledge, with the cloak of prestige lent by "objective science," has propelled the notion that one's identity is an innate, natural, and immutable quality. Gamete donation, for instance, has precipitated a return to ideas of genetic and racial essentialism, in which sperm and egg donor profiles are scrutinized for certain traits, with the promise of inheritable phenotypic and skin color characteristics, among other features. In India, the rise of consumers seeking assisted reproductive technologies has revitalized beliefs in the biological origins of caste, reifying it as a heritable biological fact rather than a social construction (Rai 2010). This resurgence has startling implications for those concerned with the feminist and bioethical issues at stake. Daniels and Heidt-Forsythe (2012), for example, show how sperm and egg donation practices in the United States reflect positive eugenic beliefs in new and more subtle forms. Reinforcing the belief that idealized (and often nonbiological) human traits are transmitted genetically, gamete donation propagates the views of the eugenics movement.

Within donor agencies there is a marked preference for matching physical characteristics, and the language of "resemblance" and "matching" serves as a neutralized proxy for race. As Thompson (2006) notes, in the case of eggs, sperm, and embryos, "the cells themselves are raced in ways that affect not just their availability and who can benefit from them, but the market value and the perceived kinship to recipients of the cells, even when detached from the donor" (2006, 548). Campbell (2007) explores these problems in the context of gamete donation in three European countries, in which governments require donated gametes to match the physical characteristics of the recipients. By analyzing the ethnic matching of gametes, Campbell argues that biology and culture are separated and then reassembled with the intention of creating offspring who resemble their parents. The meaning of race hovers over biology, inherited physical appearance, and culture, harkening back to the eugenic era though reconfigured as consumer choice. This is what Taussig, Rapp, and Heath (2008) have called "flexible eugenics."

This resurgence of genetic essentialism in the context of gamete donation has important consequences for notions of identity and belonging, because to claim a certain social identity always implies particular rights and obligations. For instance, articulating what counts as a mother-child relationship in the world of surrogacy and egg donation determines what mothers and children owe each other. As Brodwin argues, we must ask difficult questions: "[H]ow does new genetic knowledge change the ways people claim connection to each other and to larger collectivities? How, in turn, does this process change the resulting webs of obligation and responsibility: personal, legal, moral, and financial?" (2002, 326). As gamete donation has led to the increasing biologization of race, these questions are of particular import in the context of ova donation across racial and national lines.

Egg Donation Practices in India

Previous studies of surrogacy in India have focused on one Gujarati clinic that primarily accepts heterosexual married couples. In this clinic, surrogates give birth to babies that will be handed over to mainly Indian and nonresident Indian couples (though the clinic also serves a significant international clientele), and in many cases both parents are the genetic parents of the child. In cases where the commissioning mother's eggs are not viable, normally either the doctor or parents will select an Indian egg donor (Vora 2009).

In contrast, my fieldwork, based in several clinics in Mumbai, included a diverse sample of 39 commissioning parents (or 26 couples/individuals) pursuing surrogacy. Of these, the 19 couples/individuals (12 gay, 7 straight) who relied on egg donation experienced it as an intensely personal transaction. They considered skin color and nationality, among other factors, in their decisions about who would provide the genetic material for their child.[3] Donor selection proved to be one of the most stressful and agonizing aspects of their conception and kinship narratives. Surrogacy guidelines in India dictate that the surrogate may not provide any genetic material in the conception of the child; if the commissioning mother's eggs are not viable, the commissioning parents must purchase eggs from a third-party egg donor. These guidelines emerge from the view that without a genetic connection to the child, the surrogate will be less likely to bond with it and therefore have little difficulty handing it over to the commissioning parents.

As a result, for couples who pursue gestational surrogacy with donor eggs in India, donor selection typically includes choosing a "local" Indian donor or egg donor agencies outside India, which may offer a white egg donor for a higher price. Some foreign egg providers travel to India; others undergo extraction in their home countries for fertilization, freezing, and shipping to India. Typically, if they can afford the higher costs, a commissioning couple will opt to fly an egg provider to India in order to achieve pregnancy through fresh embryo transfer for an improved rate of success over frozen embryo transfer. In rare cases a couple may bring a friend or family member to India as an egg donor. Nearly all parents noted that the options for donor selection—where skin color and country of origin are prominent selection criteria—prompted difficult discussions about race, kinship, matching, and other desired physical characteristics of the child. Race, skin color, and nationality were nearly always a subtext in narratives about egg donation.

Egg providers' nationality and skin color also influenced payment, though in complicated ways. In the global spaces in which transnational surrogacy occurs, one finds intersecting ideas of race, beauty, and value, emerging in distinct ways at varying local/global scales, revealing local and transnational inequalities. For instance, white donors received higher pay than Indian donors; in my study, Indian donors typically received between U.S.$180 and U.S.$360, while white donors from South

Africa received U.S.$2,200. (By contrast agencies in the United States have been known to pay a premium to African American and Asian American egg providers because demand outstrips supply.) Yet in a global economy, egg providers of similar racial background too are differently positioned to one another in terms of their relationship to the state, power, the global economy, and ova recipients (Nahman 2008). Indeed, commissioning parents desiring white donors often opted for donors from countries in eastern Europe or from South Africa, where donor payments were significantly lower.

In this study, however, a minority of parents opted to purchase eggs from a white egg provider. Of the 19 couples/individuals who used egg donation, only 4 chose to use eggs from a white woman. Three of these couples were white heterosexual married couples, and their donors originated in South Africa, eastern Europe, and Canada; one gay male couple also opted for a white donor from South Africa. One individual (a single, white U.S. gay male) opted for an Asian egg provider from China, the country in which he was then living and working. The remaining 14 couples/individuals who used egg donation opted for Indian egg providers. Of these, the majority—10 couples/individuals—were gay males, 8 all-white and 2 mixed (one each white/Asian and white/Latino). Four heterosexual married couples also opted for Indian donors; these too were primarily white, with the exception of one African American woman (whose husband was white) (see Table 3.1).

As commissioning parents navigate the process of egg donation across racial, ethnic, and national lines, it is important to contextualize these negotiations within the transnational hierarchies in which they occur. Transnational reproduction occurs within a "racialized social structure" (Winant 2004) in which commissioning parents confront the transnational inequalities that privilege their capacities to become parents while relying on the reproductive labor of women in the global South. In this context, how do ART consumers make decisions about who will provide the genetic material for their child? As transnational egg donation involves the movement of donors, gametes, and embryos across borders, I found that doctors and commissioning parents dealt with stratification in diverse ways. In what follows, I detail the ways in which doctors organize donor profiles hierarchically along lines of class and skin color, shedding light on how parents understand and negotiate

TABLE 3.1. Characteristics of commissioning parents and their egg donors

Pseudonym	Sexual orientation	Ethnicity of commissioning couple/individual	Ethnicity of egg donor
Aaron/Ben	Gay	White	White (South Africa)
Adam/Nadine	Straight	White	White (South Africa)
Alain/Gaspar	Gay	White	Indian
Andrew	Gay	White	Indian
Carson	Gay	White	Indian
Fred	Gay	White	Asian (China)
Jan	Straight	White	Indian
Jason/William	Gay	White	Indian
Liz	Straight	White	Indian
Lucas/James	Gay	White	Indian
Mark/Lionel	Gay	White	Indian
Marla/Roland	Straight	White	White (eastern Europe)
Marlene	Straight	African-American (w/white husband)	Indian
Martin	Gay	White	Indian
Matthew/Anthony	Gay	White/Asian	Indian
Patricia	Straight	White	Indian
Sharon/Ahmet	Straight	White	White (Canada)
Simon	Gay	White	Indian
Tristan/Juan	Gay	White/Latino	Indian

this process. I show that while Indian doctors rely on kinship models that privilege whiteness, Western commissioning parents often rejected such models and opted for Indian egg providers for varying reasons.

Stratifiying Donors and Divas

I first came to realize that the system of transnational reproductive services values human eggs by the egg providers' skin color in an interview with Dr. Guha in October 2010. Dr. Guha was the managing director of a well-known agency that facilitated surrogacy arrangements between surrogates and intended parents, the majority of whom are foreign clients who travel to Mumbai from all over the world. We had met several times during the course of my research in Mumbai, and when we finally sat down to have an extended conversation about his work, the interview followed a familiar script. Like most doctors involved in the surrogacy industry, Dr. Guha always emphasized his compliance with government guidelines and transparency when it came to standards of medical practice and care. He shared his international clients' testimonials and told me how much he values making a baby and "completing a family." Like many of the doctors who provided surrogacy services, Dr. Guha shrugged off any criticism of or challenge to the ethics of his work by repeating perhaps the most important line in doctors' surrogacy script: surrogacy is a "win-win" situation for all actors involved, providing much-needed income for the families of poor women and highly desired children for infertile couples.

Toward the end of the interview, however, the conversation took an interesting and unexpected turn. As we were concluding the interview, Dr. Guha suddenly lowered his voice and said, "Now, I have a personal question I would like to ask you." He continued, "It's just a thought, so don't feel offended or anything—but we get a lot of queries for Oriental donors. *Would you like to be a donor?*"[4] Somewhat taken aback by the request and unsure I had heard him correctly, I asked for clarification and he continued, "Yes, Oriental donors. You see, the compensation we give is very different from others. We can give a compensation of more than U.S.$2,000. See, if you want a Caucasian donor or an Oriental donor, it's more worth it [to clients] if you are already here—so you don't have to fly them [donors] in to India and pay travel costs." Though he couched his inquiry in terms of the potential financial windfall to me as a prospective Asian egg donor, I quickly gathered that Dr. Guha was at least partly motivated by the prospect of offering his foreign clients the best deal he could.

I became deeply curious about the egg donation procedure. Two thousand dollars is indeed a grand sum of money in India (though a fraction of what many egg donors might receive in the United States, for example), and many times greater than what Indian egg donors I had interviewed received. I wondered: how do doctors classify their egg donors and how do they determine payment for donors of different racial and ethnic backgrounds? Who are the couples seeking "Oriental donors" and where do they come from?

As Dr. Guha told me of the many inquiries he received from couples in Hong Kong and Taiwan, as well as from Chinese or Japanese couples who live in the United States, Canada, and Australia, he turned to his computer to show me his confidential database of donor profiles. As I scanned his computer screen and debated how to decline his query, something on the screen caught my eye: two distinct categories, "Diva donors" and "regular donors" marked each profile. When I asked about this distinction, Dr. Guha responded, "Normally, the donors you would get from India are from the same background as the surrogates. They are not very educated, not very gorgeous or beautiful. . . . [Diva donors] are highly educated. She's from a 'Harvard' background. She's highly professional. Their compensation is different."

Here, Dr. Guha subtly indicated the ways in which the medical establishment determines what kinds of women are appropriate for different kinds of ART labor. While the bodies of lower-status women are deemed appropriate for surrogacy, they can also provide the genetic material used in IVF (albeit at a lower price). The eggs of higher-status women, however, are more highly valued on the market and thus receive higher compensation than "regular" women. But these women are not considered "good" candidates for surrogacy. One doctor explained the difference between working with women of different class and educational backgrounds in the following way: "The good thing is that they [higher-educated women] can read a prescription. The bad thing is they think they're smarter than you. The others will take your word as God's. With simple things, they will not shake without asking if it's ok. But the ones who think they're super smart, they'll just do whatever they want on their own." For Dr. Guha and other doctors, lower-class, uneducated women represent docile, submissive bodies, ideal for gestational surrogacy. On the other hand, upper-class women, perceived as strong-willed and insubordinate, are more suited for the shorter-term commitment of egg donation and are rarely recruited as surrogates. This problematic division of labor reinforces an unequal distribution of benefits and burdens along race and class lines.

Moreover, from the photographs that accompanied Dr. Guha's egg donor profiles I could see that the regular donors who were "not very educated, gorgeous or beautiful" were almost uniformly dressed in traditional Indian clothes, that is, a *salwar kameez* or *sari*, with simple, unsmiling mug shots. Doctors described them as having "dark" or "dark wheatish" skin color, and they typically had low levels of education, with "professions" listed as domestic work or "housewife." The diva donors' photos, on the other hand, resembled "glamour shots" one might see in a photographer's studio: the women wore heavy makeup and Western clothing (a shirt or blouse with denim jeans, for instance) and soft lighting framed their smiling faces. Moreover, all the diva donors were fair-skinned with lighter colored eyes and taller-than-average height, and they shared a range of profile characteristics including personality traits, profession, and education.

Dr. Guha's donor database commodified markers of class, race, skin color, and social status, reflecting an imagined Lamarckian transmission of acquired traits. He recruited low-income, darker-skinned Indian women as the providers of "regular" eggs, while women of higher social status provided the genetic material with highly desired characteristics. At the same time, Dr. Guha's database illustrated the organizing principles of egg donation: notions of beauty and desirability overlapped with education, class, and modernity, while his database considered the less attractive, that is, "not very gorgeous or beautiful" women who were low status and not ideal sources of genetic material for Western couples, as surrogates. Race, to be sure, is an organizing criterion for egg donation, and medical practitioners perpetually reify race as a valid classificatory system when assessing patients (Garcia 2003). Indeed, I witnessed this firsthand as Dr. Guha informed me that my own Asian/"Oriental" features could fetch high payments and a spot in the diva donor database.

These divisions also reflected regional inequalities and prejudices between north and south India. In a burgeoning surrogacy clinic in Delhi, I found that like Dr. Guha in Mumbai, Dr. Verma categorized her profiles of egg providers hierarchically. When asked to describe her clinic's database of egg providers, which, like Dr. Guha, included only Indian women, Dr. Verma began by describing the categorization of women's profiles:

> I have two categories: the A-list are highly professional, models, absolutely stunning women. I have a doctor who's an egg donor. A lecturer at a university here. They get up to U.S.$2,000. Usual egg donor compensa-

tion is around U.S.$630. See, here [turning her computer screen toward me] this is one of my A-list egg donors. She's a model. She was here in the clinic the other day and everybody in the hospital was going gaga. I have a few who are like that. You can't see but she has green eyes. That's very unusual for India. She's a university graduate. Here's another one; she's also a university graduate. Then I have some "Asian-looking" profiles; see, she's Asian-looking, so if we have an Asian-looking intended parent, they can have her.

Dr. Verma continued to show me profiles of engineering students, university graduates, and other donors with professional backgrounds, and emphasized, "Being in the north of India, you'll see that people here are different from Bombay or the south because people here have fairer complexion, sharper features. They are more smartly dressed. It's just a culture thing in Delhi. So there is a better choice of egg donors here." Eventually, she showed me a few profiles in the less desirable category, the "D-category," where the women were "uneducated, young girls."

Interestingly, caste or religion rarely surfaced in interviews with doctors or intended parents, except in my conversation with Dr. Verma. When asked whether other factors might play a role in egg donation and surrogacy, Dr. Verma disclosed, "Yes, but not for the surrogate. I had one couple who were Muslim and from a Muslim country somewhere in the Middle East. They wanted only a Muslim surrogate and a Muslim egg donor. That was the only case I've encountered." With respect to surrogacy, on the other hand, Dr. Verma indicated that caste became an issue only in relation to the health of the baby:

The only thing people might be concerned about [with respect to caste] is that in India, some higher-caste Hindus are vegetarian. They are concerned with the nutrition of the baby. So we absolutely load [the surrogate] with nutrition. There's this girl who's in charge of nutrition at the home [where surrogates stay during their pregnancies] and she has a goody bag that's filled with biscuits, vitamins, and other snacks. So it doesn't matter if they're vegetarians. Most of our babies are three kilos (about six and a half pounds). In the north, people are taller, broad-shouldered, so they are able to carry the pregnancy just fine.

Dr. Verma's comments illuminate how social hierarchies work in India. Framed in terms of "choice," Dr. Verma placed north India, and specifically the cosmopolitan city of Delhi, at the top of the list from which egg purchasers may select "A-list" eggs, due to its culture and reputation in India as well as the prevalence of people with lighter-skinned, "sharper features" less common in the south. She also underscored the role of caste in surrogacy, again highlighting regional difference as she moved from descriptions of nourishing higher-caste Hindus to claims of better physical fitness for childbearing among women in the north of India. Such practices elucidate the ways that physicians work to reinforce skin color and other physical characteristics (attributed to regional difference) as biologically inheritable; doctors, who have culturally sanctioned authority that extends to reproduction (Jordan and Davis-Floyd 1992), are in a unique position to perpetually reify skin color and other forms of difference as valid systems of classification. Here we see the salience of skin color as a classificatory system in egg donation, revealing hope for or a belief in some kind of biological persistence of skin tone (Thompson 2009).

In India, skin color matters, and donor eggs were valued in an economy of color reflective of a history of colonialism and racism. A light complexion confers symbolic capital in marriage negotiations among South Asians (Vaid 2009), and financial capital in negotiations between South Asians and prospective parents. Most doctors had separate files or databases for fair and dark-skinned donors, and as doctors' narratives illustrate, in these files skin color nearly always overlapped with education, class, and beauty (Almeling 2011).

During my fieldwork I found that other doctors crafted their presentation of their egg seller profiles in much the same way as Dr. Verma and Dr. Guha, according to their perceptions of what clients would find desirable. In many cases these profiles do indeed conform to the expectations of prospective parents who favor fair-skinned donors. Yet at the same time, I found that many intended parents did *not* explicitly desire the fair-skinned, highly-educated egg donor. Moreover, as I will discuss, parents described Indian donors in general as desirable precisely because of their Otherness or exotic beauty, where racialized perceptions of beauty both opened up a space for resistance to whiteness but also a reinforcement of racial/racist stereotypes.

"Appropriate" Matches and the Reproduction of Whiteness

Ethnographic research on egg and sperm donation indicates that prospective parents commonly seek phenotypic, personal, and cultural "matching"—seeking donors who share a similar racial/ethnic background, personal qualities, and phenotype—between egg donors and intended mother or sperm donor and infertile male partner, and agencies or doctors commonly encourage the practice (Becker 2000; Thompson 2005). Such matching appeared to keep assisted reproduction as "natural" as possible while also allowing families to be discreet and maintain secrecy regarding donor use, giving parents full control over domestic decisions about disclosure to their children about their "origin stories."

Infamous ART cases around the world reinforce this presumption of ethnoracial matching and reveal the desirability of racial purity. The media and public reaction in response to these cases is telling. In response to a 2002 case in which a white couple had mixed-race twins after an Asian man's sperm was mistakenly used to fertilize the intended mother's eggs, the woman was later quoted as saying, "All we wanted was a family. Instead we were landed with a nightmare that will last forever" (NewsCore 2012). Quiroga has noted how media accounts referred to the case of an African American woman inseminated with the "wrong" sperm (from a white man) as a "dream . . . turned into a nightmare," "unthinkable," "a fertility screw-up," and a "fiasco" (2007, 143). Drawing on such examples and her own fieldwork on gamete donation, infertility, and race in the United States, Quiroga asserts what while the stated goal of the U.S. infertility industry is to "create families," what remains unspoken is "the desire to create a certain type of family, one that closely matches, and thus reproduces, the heteropatriarchal model of a white nuclear family" (2007, 144). Quiroga ultimately argues, "ARTs' privileging of genetic relatedness is currently deployed in ways that support a white heteropatriarchal model of family in which race and whiteness are reified as inheritable" (2007, 144).

Throughout my own research, I encountered many examples of ways in which IVF, egg donation, and surrogacy in India bolstered white, heteropatriarchal kinship patterns and reflected fears about race mixing. For instance, Dr. Singh, a Mumbai-based IVF specialist, discussed her surprise at how often her clients, particularly her clients in same-sex relationships, opted for Indian donors with darker skin:

> I kept pushing the lighter skins [on same-sex couples], because I feel it's hard for a child to go through life with two dads, and then you put the child through color difference in a society. It's something that's going to bother them later. So if they do agree, I can tilt them towards, you know, "These are the options and that's what you can use, but think about it really hard before you choose a darker color skin." . . . Children do not understand racism, but they do understand color and they do understand difference, like, "Why are you so different from your parents? Why do you have two dads?"

Dr. Singh found it difficult to accept that a couple would want to conceive a child who would be a racial mismatch to its own family. Indeed, as the doctor and facilitator of surrogacy arrangements, she often used her position of authority to attempt to influence prospective parents' decisions in egg donor selection.

Although Dr. Singh found it troubling that same-sex couples in particular expressed a preference for donors with darker skin, such couples clearly have no option of concealing the use of assisted reproduction. I found, just as Dr. Singh described, that same-sex couples rarely made matching racial/skin color characteristics a high priority. While Dr. Singh described this preference for nonwhite donors or donors with darker skin tones as signaling an increased "sensitivity" and openness on the part of her gay clients, she thought that the stigma of being the child of same-sex parents should be all the more reason for same-sex parents to avoid dark-skinned donors.

Marlene Sawyer, an African American woman in her late forties and mother of a two-year-old son born through surrogacy in India, also reported that her doctor had an opinion about her taste in skin color in an egg provider. Marlene's husband is white, and they needed the assistance of donor eggs. According to Marlene: "I sent her emails and said, 'Here is a picture of me and my husband. As you can tell, I am a dark, black woman. Please give us the darkest donor you have.' What do we get? The whitest donor she has!" When I asked Marlene why she thought her doctor had taken matters into her own hands, she said:

I have no idea. I think she probably was looking at it for my husband, because my husband is a white male. So I thought maybe she was thinking, culturally or something, since the men are so dominant, "Oh, we'll give her someone that looks like her husband." I mean, I showed you the picture of Sean [Marlene's son], right? (*shows picture*). He's white as white can be.

Marlene's experience as an African American woman contrasted sharply with the majority of intended parents who traveled to India, who were white. While Dr. Singh expressed concern over the multiple boundary-crossings committed by same-sex parents who seek darker-skinned egg donors—parents who challenge heteronormative models of kinship and resist expectations to reproduce whiteness at the same time—Marlene's doctor ignored her request for a donor who matched her skin color, a move that Marlene believes has impacted her experience as a black mother. Marlene divulged, "Even though I love Sean, I don't want to feel like an outsider. Even though he never makes me feel that way, he loves me and he's my baby, I want him to get a little darker!" When I asked her about challenges or concerns that had come up for her since the birth of her son, Marlene replied:

People don't understand; they think I'm the nanny, or they say, you must be babysitting today. When little kids say it I don't care, but when adults say it, I say *I'm* his mother. And they're kind of caught off guard. I'm like, I don't have to explain Sean's existence to anyone. When Sean is of age and he wants to tell his story, he can tell his story. I feel like, as a black woman, why are you questioning me? That kind of stuff, I'm trying to figure out how to deal with it, where I'll feel comfortable.

Liz's story, like Marlene's, elucidates the problems and anxieties that stem from lack of transparency and trust in the doctors who arrange surrogacy packages from half a world away. A U.S. mother of twins born through surrogacy in India, Liz was fifty-four years old at the time of their birth. She and her husband had fourteen children, including Liz's five from a previous marriage. Their fourteenth child was adopted from Guatemala; they turned to surrogacy in India to increase their family again only after a disrupted process in Vietnam. Though Liz had heard that most doctors would only accept childless clients with histories of infertility and within a certain age range, Liz had also heard that some doctors did not adhere to this rule. After sending several inquiries and receiving multiple rejections from doctors, they found Dr. Sen in Delhi.

Because Liz was menopausal, the couple would need donor eggs in their surrogacy process. When I asked about her experience with egg donation, Liz explained:

> We were eager to have the donor be Indian as we had this idea of a sort of transworld cosmic connection through that, since we had really wanted to adopt [internationally]. We did tell them we hoped she [the egg donor] was reasonably attractive and healthy and intelligent, but we did not do any selecting, since they didn't offer it, and we knew that they would be able to select based on medical criteria. We suspect that he did not actually use an Indian donor because they stressed how they needed a picture of me to choose a suitable person, and the babies are very very fair. . . . [Dr. Sen] made mention of how he uses his best judgment on egg donors, and I got the distinct impression that he would do just what he thought best. . . . We were told just about nothing of the egg donor. John asked and was shown an indistinct photo of an Indian woman.

Liz's mistrust of Dr. Sen extended beyond her impression that he had selected an egg donor without regard for her instructions:

> He wanted LOTS of sperm samples from John, even after the day that they did the egg retrieval and fertilization for our twins. . . . It honestly never crossed either of our minds that any doctor could be so lacking in ethics to do such a thing as "borrow" other people's genetic material without disclosing that it would be given out to other strangers. I don't know how to even deal with this.

I frequently heard stories of misdeeds circulated among parents pursuing global surrogacy. In the absence of formal legislation or regulatory mechanisms regarding the use or provision of ARTs in India, parents such as Liz—who lived beyond India's borders and thus had little recourse to legal action—often resigned themselves to speculation about the source of their children's genetic material. Liz's experience also reflects issues that arose in many of my interviews with intended parents; foremost among these was the issue of trust between client and doctor, and fears about what could happen when the commercial exchange takes places across multiple geographic/cultural boundaries. Indeed, many parents spoke of the need to "blindly trust" their doctor in order to move ahead with surrogacy in India.

Marlene's and Liz's stories reflect the power that doctors hold in defining what is "desirable" in a donor and creating "acceptable" families. Like Roberts's (2012) finding that Ecuadorian clinicians frequently aimed to make whiter children through sperm and egg donation, my study too reveals how doctors view themselves as key players in a whitening project and deliberately select donors based on their lightness, regardless of what the intended parent may request.

But what motivates an intended parent to request a donor of a different racial, ethnic, or national background; or more specifically, what motivates white intended parents to select Indian egg donors? Liz's narrative reveals a common thread among intended parents who explicitly desired an Indian egg donor. Liz and her husband specifically hoped for a child who might reflect and fulfill her wish for some kind of a "transworld cosmic connection," a connection rooted in her desire for a family filled with internationally adopted children. As I will discuss in the following section, couples frequently opted to forgo ethnic or skin color matching in favor of donors from nonmatching backgrounds (phenotypic, ethnicity, race, culture, etc.). Indeed, of the 19 couples/individuals who used donor eggs, only 4 parents purchased eggs from donors of a matching (white) background. Of those who opted for eggs from Indian women, 4 couples/individuals took into account the woman's skin color, indicating a preference for fair- or dark-skinned donors, depending on the commissioning couple's own skin color. The majority (10 out of 14 couples), however, selected Indian egg donors with darker skin tones than their own. This desire reflected in part a "primordial ethnic authenticity" (Thompson 2009, 143), where expressions of desire for children who "looked Indian" were often interchangeable with expressions of desire for a child who "looked exotic." Such desires reflect the complex dynamics of reproductive tourism in which intended parents' desires for exotic-looking children are entangled with rescue narratives that frame the parents as "saving" surrogate mothers and egg providers.

The Biologization of Race, Skin Color, and Nation

While rates of compensation, doctors' practices, and beliefs about racial matching revealed the stratification of egg providers along race and color lines, in practice intended parents select egg donors based on a range of "qualifications." The process of egg donation in India differs vastly from that in the home countries of most intended parents. For instance, based on their knowledge or experience with agencies in the United States, many intended parents expected to receive, at the very least, basic information about ancestry, genetic history, as well as personality characteristics. Practitioners in India made much less information available.

In this context, what "qualifications" did commissioning parents look for? Patricia, a forty-four-year-old U.S. mother introduced in the previous chapter, would have liked to use an egg donor from a developed country but couldn't afford the higher costs. When she and her husband decided to choose an Indian egg provider, she explained how she sought more information about the women's background:

> I did actually try to develop a little questionnaire to ask our egg donors some questions, to try and find out a little more about her potential. It didn't work very well. . . . I tried to ask questions in a way to try to uncover her potential rather than her actual, things she had achieved. But it did make me aware that the circumstances that she lived in didn't really give her any possibility of exploring her potential. It was a little bit of a fruitless exercise and it made me a little bit sad, just knowing how limited her options had been. Basically we picked someone who we thought was pretty. And that's not what you ideally would want to base your decision on.

After asking her doctor to share the questionnaire with potential egg providers, Patricia recognized the social and economic constraints that limited Indian women's access to education. Thus she accepted that she had to use much simpler criteria for selection, based on beauty.

When I asked her to expand on her process of selecting the egg donor, Patricia underscored that skin color also factored into her decision:

> We picked one of the fairer egg donors that we found. There was something about her face that reminded me of people on my side of the family.

It's funny, because even my father, not knowing that, said that he [my son] looks like his brother. And that's exactly the side of the family that her face shape had reminded me of. There were a lot of factors in the looks that we considered, and definitely someone who would "blend" into our family was one of them. We were totally shocked though that he ended up having blue eyes and reddish hair! Of all the things I expected when picking an Indian egg donor, that would have been at the bottom of the list. It's just completely a genetic surprise.

Here, Patricia (like Jan, whose story opens this chapter) engaged in a kind of "resemblance talk" (Becker, Butler, and Nachtigall 2005). Patricia and Jan, among other parents in this study, recognized the cultural significance of resemblance and searched for familiar qualities in their egg donor regardless of the donor's ethnic background.

Mark and Lionel, on the other hand, an Australian Italian couple in their early thirties and parents of a son born to a surrogate mother in Delhi, ultimately settled on an Indian donor they felt was "beautiful" and evoked a kind of Indian "authenticity":

LIONEL: We received a number of profiles, which basically consisted of age, initials . . .

MARK: Some of them would have a picture and a few words, others would have all these . . .

L: . . . blank fields. We just sat there and went through and had very distinctive feelings about, "Oh, no way," and "Oh, she's so pretty," or "Oh, she likes confetti, that's quirky." But we both felt that we were attracted to a story.

M: Yeah, we said, "Can we have more information about *her*?"

L: Some of these profiles are, you know, the shots that you take when you're "Miss India," ten superhot gorgeous, over-make-upped—

M: Yeah and the background, everything is like "mistyland" or something.

L: We were like, no, we wanted something *authentic*.

M: All of JM's photos, they were just very natural. Very simple shots, and that's what we like, I guess. That's how we chose, basically. At the end of the day, it was just a sense of warmth . . . [emphasis in the original]

Lionel went on to explain their desire for an Indian donor: "We actually always thought that, because India is allowing us to do this, it was natural to have the child be . . . of India. In a way our child belongs to India. The other thing is, Lionel and I don't care what race the child is. Actually I was surprised to learn that couples were still seeking egg donors from outside of India."

Patricia, Mark, and Lionel's comments reflect those of many of the parents I interviewed, who cited a variety of reasons for selecting an Indian egg donor. While Patricia cited cost as a major factor, Mark and Lionel cited reasons that reflected an essentialized understanding of race. Despite their claim that race was irrelevant to their decision making, Mark and Lionel sought a kind of Indian "authenticity" that was "natural" and "simple." In their belief that their child was "of India," they expressed an understanding of race as a persistent biological category.

Several parents shared this conviction that genes from an Indian woman conferred an "authentic" Indian identity to the child born through egg donation and surrogacy, though occasionally couples disagreed. The story of Matthew and Anthony—fathers to three girls born through surrogacy in India—illustrates the complexities of transnational reproduction and the questions that many couples face with respect to kinship and ethnic identity. Two surrogate mothers carried the three children—twins and a singleton—who were conceived with the eggs of one Indian egg provider, and sperm samples from each father. As a result each partner was genetically related to at least one child, and the children were "connected" through a single genetic donor. Thirty-six-year-old Matthew described the complicated nature of this twenty-first century family: "Imagine the first day of school. We've got—these are triplets, in a sense, but there are different birthdays, and different fathers, but the same mother, and different last names." Interestingly, Matthew attributed motherhood status not to the surrogates who carried and birthed their children, but to the egg provider who contributed the genes in the conception of the three girls.

As Matthew and Anthony pondered what they would tell their daughters about their family's unique history, Matthew enthusiastically shared his views on his daughters' ethnic identity: "I love that our children are Indian. And that makes me a little bit Indian, too. So I want to make sure that they have a connection to their heritage. I expect we're going to go back someday. You know, I don't know when, but now India is a part of our children's heritage." However, thirty-eight-year-old Anthony heartily disagreed. Born and raised in China before moving to the United States at eighteen, Anthony claimed, "Well, the Indian part is nice, but I'm Chinese, so they're going to be more Chinese." Indeed, Matthew and Anthony chose their egg provider because, hailing from northern India, "She looked Chinese," and Anthony felt ambivalent about their children's identity as Indian. As Anthony argued that the girls would be "more Chinese than Indian," Matthew conceded his point yet noted the complexity of their family's story, reiterating, "But India is a part of our children's heritage. It's a part of our history now. And it always will be."

Martin's story further illustrates the role that skin color plays in transnational reproduction. Martin, a forty-two-year-old gay male expecting twins with his longtime partner, discussed his approach to selecting an egg provider and described the process as "the most emotional and traumatic part of the entire process." This was due in part to the lack of information available: "You have a picture, you have height and weight, and you know whether they're Hindu or Muslim. That's about it." Martin went on to explain:

> The hardest thing is you sit there and you look at these women, and you try to picture her as the mother of your child. It's so beyond even looking at her facial features and looking at her smile; it's like, do they look like a happy person? We narrowed it down to five or six that we felt fit our vision of what would be attractive. We looked for women who were relatively fair-skinned. Although we know the child's going to be part Indian, we didn't want it to come up with a really dark complexion. And it says that on the profile: fair, medium, or dark. So that was part of it for us. We also definitely intentionally chose someone who was Hindu. We intentionally did not want a Muslim. I'm Catholic and I studied religion in college and I just didn't really want that connection to Islam. And I love the Hindu faith, the deities, everything about the way they worship. I thought that, for me, I would be a lot more interested in telling my child, "This is the background that I came from, and this is the background that your mother came from," and introduce them to both and let the child select which of those they'd be interested in. I didn't know that much about Islam and I didn't really want to go down that path. We want religion to

be a big part of our children's lives and so for me, I would rather present to them those two options. And obviously if they want to go a different route, they can, but in my mind I like the idea of Hinduism.

Like many parents I interviewed, Martin ascribed motherhood status to the genetic donor, not the surrogate mother, which contributed to the stress and tension that surrounded the process of selecting an egg provider. Indeed, when I asked him what he knew about the woman who was carrying his future children, Martin replied, "Very little. And you don't typically pick the surrogate. The doctor picks her for you. I know that she has a child and that she's married, but I don't know anything more than that." While Martin described a deeper emotional investment in selecting the egg provider, the future "mother" of his children, he also revealed an emotional detachment from the surrogate, indicating the complex ways in which parents construct intimacy and intimate relations with the various reproductive actors who contribute to the conception and birth of a child. Martin, like other participants in this study, constructed a deeper intimacy with the "mother" of his twin boys, based on a genetic, not gestational, relationship.

But precisely what is transmitted through this "intimate" genetic relationship? For Martin, notions of beauty clearly overlapped with fair skin. Yet he believed that religious identity too was embedded in genetic ties. Thus he sought to circumscribe the realm of religious possibility for his children by choosing a Hindu egg provider. As I have previously argued, "understandings about a child's biogenetic origins emerge in tension with a child's right to identity" (Deomampo 2013, 530). While many parents I spoke with expressed a strong desire to "maintain the Indian element" in their children's identities, for Martin biogenetic origins also intersected meaningfully with religious identity.

Other parents, particularly white parents, articulated racialized notions of beauty in their discussions of Indian egg donation and "mixed-race" children. Marla, the thirty-two-year-old Norwegian mother of a baby girl born via surrogacy in Mumbai, explained:

Since we had to have a donor, I told Roland that I didn't mind having an Indian donor. . . . I said, "I don't mind and I know that it's good to mix races." I told him that, "It's actually not a bad thing. It's a good thing."

Indian mixes or the Indian and the white mixes that we have seen, the children are so beautiful. They are absolutely beautiful. They are lovely. So, I told him that. To me, it doesn't matter, but he wanted to try it [donation with a white donor] one time.

Though Marla claims she would have considered an Indian egg donor due to the "loveliness" and "beauty" of children of mixed descent, she ultimately decided to go with a white egg donor from eastern Europe, mostly due to her husband's desire to maintain resemblance and secrecy regarding surrogacy.

As I have discussed in this chapter, transnational egg donation encompasses multiple racial and national projects. In some cases, parents may explicitly seek to reproduce whiteness or resemblance. In other cases, however, parents sought to subvert dominant kinship models that privilege whiteness by deliberately selecting Indian egg donors that reflected notions of mixed-race beauty or a kind of Indian authenticity. Such actions, nonetheless, maintain racial/racist structures that rely on essentialized notions of culture and racialized beauty. Moreover, transnational egg donation underscores the salience of donor skin color (often conflated with race or nationality) in donor selection, even though genetic determination of skin color, among other traits, is unpredictable at best. Ultimately, as doctors and parents organize and negotiate the process of transnational egg donation, the social constructs of race, skin color, and nationality become ever more biologized within transnational relations of power.

4

The Making of Citizens and Parents

In July 2010, consuls general of eight European countries sent letters to over ten Mumbai surrogacy clinics, demanding the clinics' cooperation in ceasing to cater to their citizens. The letter, endorsed by the consuls general of Belgium, France, Germany, Italy, the Netherlands, Poland, Spain, and the Czech Republic, emphasized the importance of directing nationals from their countries to their respective consulates before beginning the surrogacy process. Moreover, the consuls general asked that clinics immediately comply with their request in order to avoid future legal hassles. Each of these countries prohibits surrogacy and many of their citizens have encountered difficulties in applying for citizenship rights for their children born via gestational surrogacy in India.

Many doctors welcomed the letter, asserting that the European consuls' general notification is in line with the Indian Council of Medical Research guidelines, which recommend that prospective surrogacy clients obtain a letter of no objection from their own consuls general (Roy 2010a). Other doctors, however, took offense to the letter. One Mumbai obstetrician conveyed her deep dismay at the thought that the dictates of foreign consulates might influence her work as an Indian doctor. When I asked how she would respond to the recent letter, she replied, "Well, I'll tell them, 'I am an Indian citizen. I follow Indian law. It allows me to do commercial surrogacy. And I don't work under you, for you. I'm not Italian, Belgian, French, whatever. So I work under my law and my guidelines.'"

These actions—of consular officials seeking to restrict their citizens' access to surrogacy in India and of doctors intent on offering surrogacy options to foreign clients—demonstrate the ways in which states and institutions become involved in transnational surrogacy, particularly when incompatible legal frameworks intersect. At the time the letter was circulated, there had been growing concern about how to deal with the legal inconsistencies that permeate the international market for surrogacy. Several high profile cases of parents unable to obtain citizenship for their babies born through surrogacy in India drew attention to the plight of "stateless babies" and to the lack of legal certainty around the connections between transnational surrogacy, nationality, kinship, and citizenship.[1]

Why were these nations intent on restricting access to surrogacy in India for their citizens? What influenced states' decisions to extend or deny citizenship to children born via surrogacy in India? At the root of these struggles for citizenship are ART consumers', providers', and state bureaucracies' conflicting ideas about race, kinship, and belonging, which are called into question in the context of the globalization of ARTs. Reproductive travelers seeking surrogacy arrangements overseas have challenged the once taken for granted correspondence between citizenship, nation, and state as new forms of citizenship take on an increasingly transnational character. Within this context, contradictory processes of citizenship—and its connections to notions of national belonging and kinship—complicate ideas about who counts as a mother, father, or parent. Moreover, even though parents and legal bureaucracies rarely mentioned race explicitly, ideas about race played a powerful role in people's negotiations with the Indian state as well as their own. In other words, the boundaries that delineate who counts as a parent and who qualifies as a citizen are deeply racialized and unstable in the context of transnational reproduction.

This chapter examines notions of citizenship and nationality in the context of transnational surrogacy, and how these notions intersect with ideas of race, kinship, and family. What happens when incompatible national legal frameworks collide in India in the process of requesting citizenship? What unfolds when different systems of kinship classification, policies about surrogacy, and practices of assigning citizenship clash—all on Indian soil? Throughout my interviews with couples and individuals who had traveled to India, I was struck by how widely their experiences varied when it came to the process of leaving India and returning home with their newest family members. I became particularly interested in the myriad ways that parents are defined—by states, institutions, and families—and how this connects with ideas and racialized practices around nationhood and citizenship. Much of the literature on the citizenship and nationality issues entangled in transnational surrogacy takes a policy or legal perspective (Ergas 2013; Points 2009); however, relatively little work engages an ethnographic approach. In what follows, I foreground the narratives of non-Indian parents of children born through surrogacy in India in order to shed light on their experiences seeking citizenship for their newborns. I focus on the citizenship process in two countries that illustrate the range of approaches to transmission of citizenship: the United States and Norway. In particular, I consider how ideas about nationhood, citizenship, family, and motherhood take on new meanings in the global lives of families built through surrogacy in India. In doing so, I argue that the process of making parents and citizens in the context of transnational reproduction simultaneously destabilizes and renaturalizes overlapping ideas about race, kinship, and belonging.

Before describing parents' encounters with the citizenship apparatus, I first situate how the domains of nationality and citizenship intersect with ideas about kinship and family. In particular, I examine the ways in which race and gender factor into such analyses of kinship and nationality, particularly within kinship models understood as being based on blood and sexual reproduction.

Racialized Practices of Citizenship, Family, and Motherhood

Historically, citizenship has been linked with the rights and obligations that individuals have within a nation-state; so too is it connected to the overall politics of belonging, as well as notions of blood and soil. As Nira Yuval-Davis and colleagues (2006) demonstrate in their work on the politics of belonging, while certain individuals and projects are seen as "belonging" within the nation-state, other individuals and projects are simultaneously excluded. But how do nations determine who does and does not "belong"?

Here, mutually reinforcing ideologies of race and nation come into play; central to these ideologies are the ways in which populations are not simply racial but racialized, through their relations and vulnerability to the state. Gilroy (1987) has noted that in postwar Britain ideas of nationality, and threats to that nationality, were strongly linked to discourses that viewed racialized immigrants (but not white immigrants) as problematic; the notion of "Britishness" was defined as white by default. Gailey (1996) has also examined the intersections between race and nationality in historical colonial context. Observing how English, French, and Dutch travelers portrayed Pacific Islanders differently at various moments, Gailey illustrates the readiness of European coloniz- ers to make judgments based on skin color. These judgments correlated with the rise of transnational slavery in West Africa and colonization in other regions. Consequently, as colonial relationships developed over the years, colonizers depicted the skin color of Pacific Islanders as no- ticeably darker.

Balibar (1991) too traces the entangled ideologies of race and nation to the moment when nation-states envision their "people" as not only political, but also as an ethnic and/or racial entity joined by a common history, origin, and culture. According to Balibar, racism and nation- alism each depend on a balance between the inclusion of citizens and people who share a common origin, and the exclusion of people out- side those categories. Racism becomes a "super-nationalism" of ideas about national culture and evokes themes of genealogical roots and purity of blood.

The origins and character of blood too have an intimate relation- ship with nationalism, and scholars have illustrated the gendered di- mensions of this relationship. While the reproduction of the nation's population involves the endless mixing of blood, the character of the individual and his/her body is seen as affected by the essence of what is inherited in the blood. Thus scholars have elucidated the ways in which ideologies of race, ethnicity, and nation, historically linked to reproduc- tive sexual relations between men and women, have a powerfully gen- dered dimension. As Stoler (1995) demonstrates, beliefs in appropriate sexual behavior and morality were central to definitions of "proper" members of the nation and the white racial category. Moreover, "ap- propriate" conduct was typically different for men and women, with women often tasked with maintaining the purity of the race, nation, or ethnic group (Smith 1997).

These notions of race and nation inevitably intersect with ideas of kinship. A starting point for this chapter is the understanding that many contemporary nation-states organize citizenship and nationality around notions of family membership. Belonging to a nation depends in part on one's belonging to a family, and several authors have linked nationalism and citizenship to ideas of kinship (Alonso 1994; Anderson 1983; Schneider 1969). Whereas in kinship, one might have relatives by blood (natural connection) and relatives by law (marriage), so too will ideologies of nationalism determine the modes of assigning citizenship: by birth or by legal process (often referred to as "naturalization"). Anderson has also argued that nationalism ought to be viewed "as if it belonged with 'kinship'" (Anderson 1983, 5).

Historically, nations have distinguished between assigning citizenship by *jus soli*, "right of the soil," or place of birth, and *jus sanguinis*, or "right of blood," in which citizenship is passed from parent to child. The principle of *jus sanguinis* in particular reiterates an unspoken blood relationship and a notion of belonging based on racial and cultural homology. This principle forms the basis of several European countries, including Norway. Yet transnational surrogacy prompts reevaluation of the importance of soil and territory. India, for instance, historically has sought to weaken claims to citizenship based on *jus soli*, in reaction to increasing numbers of undocumented migrants to the country. But in response to recent claims of babies left "stateless" in India as a result of surrogacy, foreign nationals have called for reconsideration of state policies that deny Indian citizenship to children born through surrogacy. These categories of blood and soil are unstable and are historically constructed.

In the context of ARTs, soil and blood are not always interlinked. Teman (2010) has shown how citizenship and motherhood mutually inform each other, particularly in the context of ARTs. In her study of surrogate motherhood in Israel, Teman examines motherhood and nationality to show how an Israeli surrogate gives birth not only to a new Jewish citizen but also to a gendered citizenship (that of the Jewish mother). Through this process, surrogacy reaffirms both the goals of nation building and a particular construction of motherhood based on ethnic lineage (wherein one is considered Jewish only if one has a Jewish mother). Surrogacy arrangements in Israel, then, are carefully managed to support the core categories of motherhood and family while achieving the reproductive goals of the state. However, as I demonstrate, conflicting laws with respect to surrogacy and assisted reproduction reflect the ways in which states delimit "acceptable" and "unacceptable" ways of building the nation, shaping how parents navigate processes of citizenship and kinship in transnational spaces.

Finally, while the concept of "citizen" has been classically defined as the legally recognized subject or national of a state, recent anthropological work on citizenship has problematized this, viewing citizenship as a mechanism through which people make different kinds of political claims. Aihwa Ong's (1999) concept of flexible citizenship, for instance, delves into the realm of the transnational, connecting global mobility and flexibility with the logics of displacement. This linkage can be applied to assisted reproduction as well. Reproductive workers such as egg donors and surrogates frequently travel long distances to participate in reproductive tourism, yet most of them are nameless, their anonymity underlining the disposability of their bodies while highlighting their biogenetic value. To discuss how transnational surrogacy complicates understandings of citizenship and kinship, and how these overlap with ideologies of race and nation, I now contrast citizenship policies and practices in India, the United States, and Norway.

Ties That Bind: Privileging Genes in U.S. Citizenship

For foreign parents who pursue surrogacy in India, the themes of citizenship and nationality are paramount. Parents often describe the process of obtaining citizenship for their children as stressful, bewildering, and maddening. In many cases the relative ease (or difficulty) with which parents undergo this process depends largely on their country of origin. Their wide-ranging encounters with state bureaucracies too indicate the multiplicity of ways in which states define citizenship and kinship.

In India, citizenship is not immediately assigned to children born in the country; instead, at least one parent must be an Indian citizen in order for the child to be Indian as well. Moreover, individuals born after 2004 are considered Indian citizens only if both parents are citizens, or if one parent is a citizen and the other is not an "illegal migrant." However, in the age of assisted reproduction questions of who the "parent" is abound. In the context of gestational surrogacy, Indian doctors and policy makers insist that the woman who contributes her own eggs to the creation of embryos (i.e., is the genetic mother of the child) and intends to raise the child is the mother of that child. In cases involving egg donation, the commissioning mother is considered the mother. Thus, according to the ICMR guidelines, the Indian surrogate who gestates and gives birth to the child (to whom she has no genetic relationship) holds no rights as a "parent" to this child. Consequently, she does not have the power to transmit Indian citizenship to the newborn. This definition of "parent," then, enables the genetic and/or commissioning parents to seek citizenship for their babies in their home countries.

These guidelines largely facilitate the transmission of citizenship for U.S. parents of children born in India. U.S. citizenship is conferred through a mixture of *jus soli* and *jus sanguinis*, in which individuals may acquire citizenship either through birth in the United States or through transmission from a U.S. citizen parent to their genetic child. Thus, for children of U.S. parents born in India, the claim to citizenship is based on a genetic connection to the parents, their U.S. citizenship, and various transmission requirements, including the parents' physical presence in the United States.

The U.S. application for citizenship for children born abroad entails a number of steps. Parents first apply for a Consular Report of Birth Abroad (CRBA), which is the primary evidence of U.S. citizenship to be used throughout the child's life for any event that normally requires a U.S. birth certificate. Along with the CRBA application, parents submit a passport application and photos. Once these applications are approved, parents must obtain an exit permit for their child from the Foreigners Regional Registration Office (FRRO), an office of India's Bureau of Immigration, in order to leave the country. In general, the CRBA, passport, and exit visa applications are time consuming and document intensive. For straightforward cases, the process can take two to three weeks; more complicated cases can take months.

With the rise of consumers seeking ART services abroad, the U.S. Department of State sought to clarify the steps needed to transmit citizenship. In 2009 the American Citizen Services Unit (ACS) in Mumbai issued a letter detailing the process for CRBA applicants who relied on surrogacy and/or gamete donation for the creation of their children. This letter emphasized the importance of "biological ties," requiring "clear evidence of the child's biological relationship to the transmitting US citizen parent." The letter and Consulate practices, however, consistently conflated biology with genetics. While the Consulate recommended carefully documenting all medical procedures in order to establish the facts of "biological parentage," its aim was to establish genetic ties, insofar as consular officers request DNA testing as verification of parentage.

These recommendations, moreover, left open some room for interpretation. In interviews with ACS staff stationed in Mumbai, officers tasked with evaluating the CRBA applications confirmed that they looked for "clear and convincing evidence" of a genetic relationship between the U.S. parent and the child. But how do officers determine what constitutes "clear and convincing" evidence? When I posed this question, officers explained that the types of documentation they receive have changed over the years. When surrogacy first came to their attention around 2007, the documentation of biological ties, such as a letter from the hospital in which the child was born, was considered unreliable but often accepted. Brad, an officer who adjudicated CRBA applications in Mumbai, remarked: "The process is awfully discretionary . . . but if it feels right, you know." When I asked him to expand on how he knows when it "feels right," he simply replied that the process is about whether "someone coming in off the street can convince you that this is your biological child." His supervisor, Carla, agreed: "You kind of have to common sense it. If you have two people come in and they both claim to be donors and they're both American citizens, they have documentation that shows that they're both in a clinic going through some procedure—and the kid's blonde! (laughs)—then, of course, it's more likely that DNA tests won't be necessary." In the absence of clear and convincing evidence, they request DNA testing.

Yet what counts as "clear and convincing evidence" is left to staff workers to decide. Although race is never explicitly discussed, the importance of racial likeness is implied, given popular assumptions regarding genetics, biological inheritance, and the heritability of race. Indeed, Carla's comment illustrates the ways in which ACS officers attach meaning to phenotype-qua-race, for instance, as it may serve to racially liken or distance parents from children. It also indicates the ways in which race is understood to overlap with nationality. The United States's history of citizenship illustrates the ways in which citizenship has been tied to race, and explicitly to whiteness (Glenn 2002). Here it manifests again, as a presumably white child with blonde hair "convinces" the officer of her "Americanness." That she might be considered Indian, on the other hand, is dismissed as implausible.

At the same time, Brad's comments illustrate the ways in which citizenship processes are historically and socially contingent. Particularly in the context of assisted reproduction, which challenges cultural and legal notions of kinship and relatedness, citizenship practices are continually in flux. Indeed, U.S. citizens' encounters with the citizenship apparatus reflect the ways in which assisted reproduction in global contexts challenges bureaucratic norms. In this context, race plays a role to varying degrees in U.S. parents' pursuit of citizenship for their children born in India.

As a result, some parents found the process straightforward while others encountered difficulties along the way. When I first met Marlene, a U.S. mother of a two-year-old son born in India, she and her husband had recently contracted with the same surrogate for a second attempt, hoping to produce a sibling for her son. Now that she was in the midst of another surrogacy process, I asked Marlene what differences she had noted between the two experiences thus far. Her main concerns, she replied, dealt with the exit process: "The first time I was worried about how long it would take to leave the country, what the protocol was, how much I was going to have to pay off people to get my son out. Now that I've done that already, I'm not worried. I already know how it's going to go." She went on to describe her experience after the birth of her son:

> At the time you had to contact the embassy to get an appointment, and the embassy said they would get us an appointment a couple weeks out. I was like, that's not happening. Number one, I said, I'm Jewish and my son needs to be circumcised. Even though I'm not! So we get there and we get this person who's just hemming and hawing, and I'm like, look, if you think I'm spending one more day here in India, think again, it's not happening. Passport was done that day. I said I want an emergency passport, because he must be circumcised. I got an emergency passport.

While many parents acknowledged the frustrations involved in the bureaucratic processes of applying for citizenship and exit visas, Marlene admitted she was proud of the way she had navigated the system to her advantage. Yet her comments also make visible one of the main perceived challenges of parents awaiting travel documents: simply having to exist in India. Marlene, like other parents, described the urge to do all that was possible so that they did not have to "spend one more day" in India, revealing their thoughts on being in India with all the discomforts it entails. The issue of comfort and discomfort is a recurring theme in many parents' accounts, divulging echoes of neocolonial views of India (and the developing world) as a site of disorder, poverty, and backwardness. Marlene also signals parents' ideas of belonging—rhetorically positioned as resting with her home country. She situates the United States as the place where she can return to the routines of everyday life, which allow her to "kin" the children as "hers."

Moreover, Marlene's son was conceived with her husband's sperm and an Indian woman's eggs. Marlene herself had no genetic connection to her son and she was traveling by herself without her husband, the sole parent who had a genetic relationship to the child. Yet she reported that the consular officer did not request a DNA test. Somehow, Marlene was able to negotiate U.S. bureaucratic processes in a way that allowed her to leave the country expeditiously and without requiring additional evidence such as DNA testing. Despite U.S. citizenship laws that reinforce genes and biology as necessary for children born abroad, the particular moment in which she sought citizenship revealed the elasticity of visa processes.

However, even as Marlene received all the necessary documents from the U.S. Consulate and the Indian FRRO, she encountered problems with airline officials at the airport as she tried to leave India:

> I didn't even think I was going to leave India. They [the airline officials] were acting like I had a stolen baby, even though I had all the paperwork. They harassed me for a good two hours—with an infant! I would never fly that airline again. They claimed that they knew nothing about surrogacy, nothing. How did I get in the country at nine months' pregnant and have a baby? I had all the paperwork, but I thought I was stuck.

Clearly, Marlene's experience of obtaining citizenship and exit documents for her son unfolded relatively simply, particularly in comparison with other parents I interviewed in similar situations who endured long delays and frustrating encounters with bureaucratic officials. Yet her position as a woman who became a mother through the use of ARTs raised questions among airline officials in India. Here it is worth noting that Marlene struggled with issues of race and racism, as Marlene is African American and her son, conceived with his white father's sperm and a fair-skinned egg donor, had much lighter skin. Paradoxically, while U.S. officials deemed Marlene's son a legitimate U.S. citizen through presumed biological connections, Indian airline officials challenged Marlene's motherhood status to a child of a different skin color than herself.

Other U.S. parents related different stories about the process of leaving India with their newborns. In her narrative, Patricia, the U.S. mother of a one-year-old son born via surrogacy in India, elucidates distinct challenges and frustrations involved in the citizenship and exit process. In order to facilitate the process and avoid long delays, Patricia studied and researched all the requirements while preparing the necessary documents. She related, "This is one area where I felt like I spent nine months totally trying to get everything perfect, to have all the paperwork printed out, to know exactly which offices to go to and when. I felt like I had researched everything and we were going to just speed through the process." However, on arrival in India, Patricia realized, "Everything was more complicated than we thought." She went on to describe the process of obtaining citizenship for her son, Sam, as a "kind of torture. In retrospect it was only two and a half weeks, but it felt at the time so long, so uncertain, it felt like we were trapped in a 'Waiting for Godot' situation."

Patricia saw her plans unravel at various moments in the process. Sam was born in mid-2009. At the time, many parents reported that like Marlene, they had been able to obtain their citizenship and travel documents without a DNA test. Patricia hoped she and her husband might avoid this additional hurdle. However, their adjudicator at the Consulate requested laboratory proof that her husband, Jonas, was the father. Patricia and Jonas assumed that their doctor would be able to provide this evidence:

> We called them [the doctors] up and we sat in the U.S. embassy office for literally eight hours waiting for the doctors to fax over proof that Jonas was the sperm donor for our son. And we had numerous conversations

with the doctors, back and forth, and what they ended up faxing over was basically a note that they had written that day. It wasn't laboratory proof, basically. So we ended up having the DNA test and we missed our appointment [with the adjudicator to apply for the CRBA].

Patricia went on to explain the communication issues embedded in her interactions with the doctors:

> It was just a whole series of stressful situations that we didn't really need to go through if we had just gone over to the doctor's office and gotten the DNA test. That was one thing that we subjected ourselves to that we probably should just have not bothered with. There was this total miscommunication. We were speaking the same language as the doctors, but we didn't feel like they understood. That was a common thing with our interactions with them. We were all speaking the same language but not quite understanding each other.

Problems of miscommunication also affected Patricia and Jonas's experience getting the Indian birth certificate, a crucial document in the process of obtaining citizenship and travel documents. The process of transnational surrogacy involves many layers of midlevel brokers, agents, and "fixers" who take care of various tasks. Patricia hired one such agent to help obtain the birth certificate, as she had heard from other parents that the Indian birth certificate office "was not a place for Westerners to go, because it was not set up to handle Westerners."

Patricia's observations indicate the ways in which culture stands in for race. She points to the ways her interactions with the doctors were fraught with miscommunication despite the fact that both parties spoke the same language. Here, she understands culture to be a sign of difference that is nearly impossible to negotiate. As Khiara Bridges states, culture can be understood as information on individual racial thoughts and fantasies, to the extent that it has become more acceptable to "talk culture," while "talking race" is disparaged (2011, 136). In other words, individuals find it easier and more acceptable to discuss difference in terms of culture than race, even though beliefs in Indian "culture" can be as harmful as beliefs in an immutable Indian "race." Moreover, Patricia's comment that the FRRO was "not set up to handle Westerners" implies a sense of chaos and disorder that has characterized representations of the global South. Such representations assume a racial character that perpetuates mainstream notions of the global South as a place of confusion, chaos, and irrationality. In this context, the global North is continually constituted vis-à-vis the South, as a space of modernity, efficiency, and competency.

Despite her best efforts to expedite the process, Patricia learned that her doctors at the surrogacy clinic became angry when she hired an agent unrelated to the clinic to take care of the birth certificate:

> We took this agent with us to the birth certificate office, and that made our doctors very pissed off. Apparently he caused some waves that made them look bad. When we got to the office the birth certificate wasn't ready, so when we got there we were looking around for someone we could bribe to get the certificate. I think after this whole experience the clinic actually started using this guy as the conduit to the birth certificate office, but at the time they were very antagonistic toward us for using him and they were yelling at us. We spent another day just basically sitting in this waiting room not really understanding what was happening or why things were not going as smoothly as we thought they would. We were there around the time when swine flu was getting big news, so we were sitting there with crowds of Indian people and a week-old baby in our arms, and it was pretty stressful.

Themes of comfort and discomfort emerged again in Patricia's remarks, echoing Marlene's desire to exit India as quickly as possible. For Patricia, India was marked as a place of disease and danger; indeed, she referred to the stress of simply being among "crowds of Indian people" with a newborn, feeling out of place and fearing the swine flu.

The birth certificate itself, however, was also a source of disappointment and stress for Patricia:

> When we started this whole process, the clear implication was that my name would be on the birth certificate. And I think at some point, as more people started to use this process [surrogacy], the U.S. embassy became stricter about how that process worked. When we called the embassy to make the appointment for the CRBA, I told them I was the ge-

netic mother. But in between then and the appointment I realized that I have absolutely no proof for that. And I don't want to get caught in a lie with the U.S. government, so we ended up going back and just my husband's name is on the birth certificate. And so the implication of that is that now I have to go through an adoption process with my son.

For many parents the process of acquiring a valid birth certificate was central to gaining citizenship rights for their child. In acquiring this document, however, many parents, like Patricia, observed firsthand the contradictions involved in the process. Indian policies define Patricia, the woman who commissioned the surrogacy process, as Sam's mother. Yet hoping to avoid any hassles in gaining U.S. citizenship for Sam, Patricia opted to withhold her name on Sam's birth certificate as his mother. Many parents believed this process was unjust and discriminatory, as commissioning parents then had to go through the process of adopting "their own children."

Interestingly, in both Marlene's and Patricia's cases, India defined them as the mothers of the children they commissioned. Yet ACS officers applied the U.S. guidelines of assigning citizenship differently to each of the women, illustrating the pliability of state citizenship practices and the ways in which states attempt to keep up with technological advances that reshape social and reproductive lives. Ultimately, these practices reinforced a reliance on genetics, renaturalizing state definitions of parenthood. As I will describe in the following section, this process takes on particular gendered dimensions in Norway.

Birth Mothers Only: Norwegian Citizenship and the Dictates of Motherhood

In the previous section I elaborated U.S. practices that value biogenetic notions of parenthood in the transmission of citizenship from parent to child, which are in line with Indian policies regarding definitions of parenthood in the context of ARTs. In contrast, Norway defines the mother solely as the woman who gives birth to the child, thus excluding any possibility that an infertile woman who intends to raise the child (and who may or may not be genetically related to the child) can be the mother without undergoing the process of adoption.

Norway's laws on the use of ARTs shed some light on this policy. Despite its reputation as a liberal, progressive country, Norway passed some of the strictest ART laws in Europe. Commercial surrogacy, egg donation, and anonymous sperm donation are all banned. As a result, infertile Norwegians frequently travel to other countries such as the United States and India (for surrogacy), Spain (for egg donation), and Denmark (for anonymous sperm donation) (Hammerstad and Haugdal 2010). What is interesting about these laws is the centrality of the role of genes and biology in the making of the Norwegian mother. Because the laws emphasize the importance of knowing one's genetic roots, anonymous sperm donation is prohibited while known sperm donation is permitted. Yet egg donation is completely banned, in part to ensure that blood and biogenetic relations remain intact, avoiding any uncertainty about who the mother may be.

These laws have important implications for notions of belonging in Norway, where the *jus sanguinis* principle—in which citizenship is transferred between parent and child—predominates. If Norwegian citizenship is attributed to children of a Norwegian birth mother, her husband, or a Norwegian man genetically related to the child, a Norwegian man, then, who uses his own sperm in the production of embryos and commissions a surrogate to gestate the fetus for him can transmit his citizenship to his children because the child is considered his genetic offspring. In contrast, a Norwegian woman who uses her own eggs and also commissions a surrogate cannot gain Norwegian citizenship for the child. Nationality is embedded in Norwegian semen, while Norwegian eggs are positioned as "belonging" to the Norwegian birthing mother alone (Kroløkke 2012). Moreover, this principle adds a gendered component to the idea that "blood is thicker than water," reiterating an unspoken blood relationship that has also functioned to ensure racial and cultural homology in Norway (Brochmann and Seland 2010).

The Norwegian focus on shared genes and biology sheds light on issues related to assisted reproduction and immigration in Norway. Interestingly, the revised 2006 Norwegian citizenship law reinforced the *jus sanguinis* principle, making requisite a shared biogenetic connection for citizenship regardless of the child's birthplace in Norway or overseas (Kroløkke 2012). Consequently, the children of noncitizen immigrants on Norwegian soil are denied citizenship, which is grounded in essentialist ideas of sameness, racially as well as culturally. In effect, biology, maternity, and citizenship overlap with racial likeness in the Norwegian context .

As a result, transnational surrogacy in India has posed particular problems for Norwegian women seeking to obtain Norwegian citizenship for their children.[2] While Indian policies effectively strip the surrogate of any parenthood rights, Norway only recognizes the birth mother—here, the Indian surrogate—as the legal mother to the child born via surrogacy arrangements. Consequently, Norwegian parents of children born through surrogacy must obtain a statement from the surrogate mother consenting to the transfer of all her parental rights to the commissioning individuals. The process of obtaining citizenship was significantly longer for Norwegians than it was for those from the United States, and I had several opportunities to interview Norwegian parents, such as Paul and Astrid, during their extended stays in Mumbai.

Paul and Astrid were thirty-four and thirty-six years old, respectively, when I met them at a restaurant in their hotel. Astrid had a high school level education, while Paul had completed university. The couple had been together since they were teens, when Astrid was seventeen and Paul fifteen, and they were married three years prior to our interview. Paul and Astrid knew that when the time came to begin thinking about raising a family together, they would turn to ARTs. As the couple explained, Astrid had received a cancer diagnosis when she was only an infant, which required her to undergo a hysterectomy (though her ovaries functioned normally). When they were ready to raise children, they began exploring their options and considered adoption. As Astrid stated, "I always thought that if I'd have children when I grow up, it would be by adoption." However, they were quickly discouraged by the low rates of domestic adoption in Norway and the long waiting periods for international adoption.

Paul and Astrid then learned about surrogacy. At first, it took some time to get used to the idea. As Astrid remarked, "If it's possible to give me hormones and take my egg out and then take sperm and put it into a petri dish—," Paul finished her thought: "It's like magic!" Surrogacy, however, is not permitted in Norway, so they knew they would need to journey abroad. Eventually they decided to travel to India, and on their third attempt their surrogate mother became pregnant with twins, conceived with frozen embryos created with Paul's sperm and Astrid's eggs. The newborn twins—one girl and one boy—slept nearby in a bassinet as the couple went on to describe their experience navigating the Norwegian citizenship process.

As Paul explained, the law is somewhat unclear regarding traveling abroad for surrogacy. Until recently, the process was fairly simple and state authorities typically accepted birth certificates without hassles. "When they started, it was not an issue at all. It was—you go here, you get the birth certificate in your names, of course, as you are the biological parents, or simply because you are the intended parents. So, Norway would just accept that birth certificate." However, with the increase in couples traveling to India from Norway for surrogacy, Paul noted, the process had become much more complicated:

> When this became an issue just a few months ago, there were several couples here, and I know it sounds incredible, but someone in government decided that there were these cases where our law needed to be clarified and no guidelines have been made. But instead of continuing the existing practice until those guidelines existed, he just stopped everything. So, they [the parents] were just stuck here without knowing how, if, or when they were going home. They were stuck here for weeks.

As Paul and Astrid awaited their own children's travel documents, Paul expected that they would not have to wait as long, given what he believed was a straightforward case:

> Fortunately, our case is very clear, and it's one of the cases that is clearly within the guidelines. We had to go to the consulate with the surrogate mother and, since she's married, she also had to bring her husband because he is assigned fatherhood by default. Because of the "pater est rule," that's who the father is. Basically, the woman is married, she has a child, and her husband is, by default, the father. So, he had to agree that I was the father, and there are then simple forms for us to fill out. So it's just a matter of filling out the forms, reassuring that she agrees and he agrees that I am the father.

Paul and Astrid's case was relatively clear because they were a married couple and each of them had a genetic tie to the children. However, the "pater est rule," as Paul stated, is a Norwegian law based on Roman principles that the woman giving birth is the mother. He continued, "Of course, that principle was intended to protect the biological mother, the genetic mother, so no one could lay claim to her children. But the presumption behind the law is that the woman giving birth is also the genetic mother, which isn't always the case anymore." Thus, according to Norwegian law, Astrid is not considered a mother to her genetic offspring and must adopt the children on her return to Norway.

As part of the process, Paul had to provide DNA evidence of his genetic relationship to the twins. At the time of our meeting he had already submitted this test to the administrative office in India that processes the citizenship applications. Yet the information must pass through multiple channels across national borders, and Paul explained that the test results needed to be sent to Norway before they could complete the process. Already into their third week in India, Paul expressed his impatience at the impending delays:

> The papers were filled out more than two weeks ago, but they still haven't left the embassy, actually, because they are extremely inefficient and slow. They insist on sending it [to Norway] by diplomatic mail, which only goes once a week. Of course, I don't know if they actually want to complicate the process, if that's their orders or what, they won't say, but they insist on sending it by diplomatic mail. And it wasn't sent the first week because they were missing an original, and they wanted the original document, not the copy. I don't know if that's really relevant for the rest of the process, but they insisted that they have the original. I don't know if that was just a cover, but they got the original and then it was just too late for it to be sent that week, so it's stuck another week, and they still haven't sent it.

As they were completing the paperwork, Paul and Astrid learned that Norwegian officials had begun enforcing a three-week waiting period for the issuance of passports following approval of the application. Paul interpreted these events as intentional efforts by the Norwegian government to stall the process for parents of children born via surrogacy: "It's extremely frustrating, to be treated in that way by our own government. When they have the DNA test, they have every reason in the world to give you the passport and just get you home. Still, they resist until the very, very last moment. So we feel that we are not treated very well. They should protect our interests and we don't feel like they are doing that at all."

Paul's interpretation of his government's actions illustrates a twist on the usual portrayals of Indian bureaucracy as rife with inefficiency. Instead, he views his nation's bureaucracy as unprofessional and disorganized, and feels that they are being treated like noncitizens by his "own government." In effect, during this liminal moment in their surrogacy journey, as they await the documents that would allow them to return to Norway, Paul calls attention to what he views as differential and discriminatory treatment due solely to the fact that they dared to travel to India—straining Norwegian dictates of "blood is thicker than water"—to have children.

In addition, Paul and Astrid's experience illustrates the challenges parents encounter in the process of gaining citizenship for their children. While the requirements for citizenship may appear clear at the outset, the guidelines and protocols are in flux and many parents endured long waits and unexpected delays. Like Paul and Astrid, another Norwegian couple I met, Marla and Roland, felt frustrated with the uncertainty of the process. Both couples' narratives illustrate the ways in which transnational surrogacy destabilizes notions of kinship and motherhood, particularly within the context of cross-border movement of people, information, and reproductive body parts. This global mobility creates a new interconnectedness—as well as new families—beyond nation-state borders. Here, kinship and citizenship processes occur throughout multiple spaces of hotels, hospitals, and bureaucratic offices, revealing global linkages and shaping social relations in transnational spaces.

When I first met Marla, a tall, blonde-haired, blue-eyed woman from Norway, she was relaxing poolside in the company of her husband, Roland, and their newborn baby girl, Anna. It was a warm, humid day in 2010 and I was visiting their deluxe, five star hotel in the suburbs of Mumbai. Marla and Roland, thirty-two and thirty-one years old, respectively, had been trying to have a child for several years before they discovered surrogacy in India. After three failed IVF attempts, they learned that because Marla suffered from a chronic disease that affected her ability to conceive and carry a child, they would have to explore other options for expanding their family. She was heartbroken by the realization, following her last attempt at IVF: "I was so sad after failing again. Well, not failing, but, you know, not working. First you are told that you can't carry a pregnancy. Then, your eggs are not working. And all the things that you are supposed to do as a woman in life . . . you're failing on all of them."

Because surrogacy is illegal in Norway, Marla and Roland's journey to parenthood led them to India, where they found a surrogacy clinic that was well known for its relationships with international clients. They decided to purchase eggs from a egg donor agency in eastern Europe, as Roland preferred to use eggs from a white egg donor. As Marla explained, "He said that it would be a lot easier for us to explain to governments and a lot of neighbors—everyone—if she's white." Though Marla had indicated that she would have been receptive to the idea of using eggs from an Indian egg provider, Roland's comment makes sense in the context of Norway, where racialized physiognomy signals cultural difference (Howell and Melhuus 2007). Consequently, embryos made from an eastern European woman's eggs and Roland's sperm were transferred into the womb of a surrogate mother in Mumbai. The resulting child, Anna, was born at a healthy 7.2 lbs via cesarean section.

I learned through my interview with the couple that their long history of medical infertility—as well as restrictive laws that made surrogacy illegal in Norway—led them to pursue surrogacy in India. Yet their journey was not over, and they were going on their fourth week in the hotel. While they were hopeful they could return home to Norway soon, they knew that realistically they could expect at least several more weeks of legal limbo while they awaited the documents that would verify their baby's citizenship and allow them to return to Norway. Marla was relishing her new role as a mother, stopping frequently during our interview to check on Anna. Yet she expressed her deep frustration with the fact that her motherhood role was illegitimate in the eyes of the Norwegian state. She spoke with anger and disbelief at the seemingly endless bureaucracy of paperwork and DNA tests that established a genetic link between father and daughter—the link that mattered, in this case, in the family's quest to return home. As she explained the process of gaining

Norwegian citizenship and travel documents for her child, she said she resented the fact that once home, she still would not be considered a mother under Norwegian law:

> Once we get all the paperwork we can go home. . . . I still will not be considered a mother in Norway because they know that it's a surrogate birth. . . . If you don't give birth to a child yourself, you are not considered a mother. It's about who is the father, and, you know, anyone can become a father if the mother of the child wants them to be. She can just point to whoever she wants to point to, and if she's married, the husband has just to sign a paper saying, "No, I'm not the father; he is." That's how you become a father. It's discriminating.

I asked Marla to expand on how she felt about this, and she replied:

> Horrible, horrible. If something happens to her in Norway, she is considered a child with only the father. If he's working, and say, she needs to go to the hospital, if they really want to be assholes at the hospital, they can say, "But you are not the mother. So, we are not allowed to give you any information about her health."

Assisted reproduction allowed Marla to move from a space in which she felt a failure—as a woman who desperately wanted to become a mother—to another space, located in India, in which she finally became one. However, though like Astrid she is considered the mother according to Indian policies, Norwegian law dictates that she is not the legal mother of her child. While Astrid held a genetic connection to her child and Marla did not, neither woman enjoyed legal motherhood rights and both would have to undergo the process of adoption on their return to Norway. Their quest for Norwegian citizenship for their children effectively reinforced notions of national belonging based on racial homology while simultaneously challenging cultural ideas about the intersection of race and motherhood in Norway.

In this chapter, I have examined particular ways in which assisted reproduction in India challenges notions of kinship and citizenship. The transnational movement of reproductive tissues and bodies clearly calls into question understandings of citizenship and motherhood. As families like those discussed in this chapter take issue with their countries' definition of motherhood and family, nations must decide how to respond to citizenship disputes in the context of transnational reproduction. Yet while such movements may expand conventional understandings of kinship and family, they also renaturalize state definitions of citizenship and motherhood. In the case of the United States, genes are framed as powerful entities that shape human relationships and confer citizenship rights and responsibilities. The same holds true in Norwegian law, although genetics and gestation are intertwined in the definition of motherhood. A Norwegian woman who does not give birth to a child, even if she is genetically related to that child, has no rights as a mother and no power to confer Norwegian citizenship on the child. These cases illustrate the evolving ways in which ARTs challenge notions of the reproductive body, citizenship, motherhood, and nation.

5

Physician Racism and the Commodification of Intimacy

I first met Dr. Singh in early 2010 at Origins Gynecology Clinic in south Mumbai. Dr. Singh had started the clinic's IVF unit three years earlier and had built a small but growing global surrogacy program. Our fifth meeting, on a cool monsoon day in August, occurred at a new clinic she had started in the northern suburbs of the city that specialized in transnational surrogacy. Eden Hill Medical Center, a quaternary care hospital offering advanced levels of specialized care as well as medical tourism services to international patients, hosted the clinic.

Dr. Singh explained that her new clinic's surrogacy program occupied much of her time. She spoke with passion about the challenges of starting her own clinic, and eventually our conversation turned to her management of the relationships between surrogates and commissioning parents. Dr. Singh believed that one of her key responsibilities was to mediate the vast geographical and social distance between surrogates and clients (commissioning parents)—parties who may never meet but nevertheless are engaged in making a baby together. I knew that she discouraged parents and surrogates from meeting, and when I asked her to explain this, she replied:

> It depends on the parent actually. Some of them want to meet. But actually I feel that until the baby is out, it's better for the surrogates not to meet the clients, because you're giving that little chance for emotional blackmail. . . . There was this whole blackmail issue [at another clinic] where the surrogate demanded some ten lakhs [around U.S.$21,000] before the cesarean. That makes me think: Why should you even give her the chance to ask? Once you see white skin and you see that they have money, it's all [claps hands]—the whole battle is lost.

Dr. Singh made explicit the relationship between the business transaction built into surrogacy and the actors' skin color and socioeconomic backgrounds when she said that once the surrogates "see white skin and that they have money," the battle against blackmail is lost. By making whiteness synonymous with commissioning clients, she recognized that surrogate and client are racialized figures. Surrogates became, by definition, nonwhite. By emphasizing what she viewed as immutable difference between surrogates and commissioning parents, Dr. Singh simultaneously highlighted the alterity of surrogates. Her statements illustrate the ways in which Indian doctors racialize the actors involved in surrogacy to justify discouraging contact between clients and surrogates.

Parents and surrogates shared Dr. Singh's sense that doctors have a central role in coordinating surrogate-client relationships at the heart of gestational surrogacy, though many commissioning parents and some surrogates told me they wished they could meet one another. This chapter therefore provides an in-depth examination of the key role that doctors play as a necessary part of illuminating the relationship between surrogates and intended parents. Thus, this chapter unfolds two interrelated analyses: first, I explore the ways in which doctors organize and facilitate surrogates' relationships with intended parents. Second, I examine how this influences the ways in which surrogates themselves understand and negotiate these relationships. Ultimately I argue that Indian doctors racialize surrogates—whose caste and class backgrounds are distinct from those of the doctors—in ways that justify their unequal position in surrogacy arrangements. I contend that these forms of racialization powerfully shape how surrogates view and experience their relationships with commissioning clients and the fetuses they bear.

Central to this chapter is the context in which surrogates and intended parents rarely, if ever, meet in person. This contrasts with the conditions that hold in previous studies of gestational surrogacy, in which parties expected some level of mutual engagement and often had a shared cultural background or at least nationality (Teman 2010; Ragoné 1994). In the United States, most surrogacy agencies encourage the intended parents to meet with their surrogate several times prior to birth, although most contact is limited to e-mail and the telephone due to the sheer geographical distance between them (Ragoné 1994). Israeli surrogacy relationships, on the other hand, rarely involve a distance of more than two hours' travel time, and the parties typically have frequent meetings as well as regular contact by phone or e-mail (Teman 2010). In India, Amrita Pande's (2014c) case study of commercial surrogacy examined how Indian surrogates constructed kinship ties with the intended parents, even when their clients traveled from countries outside India. Yet even across vast geographical distances, doctors in Pande's study ensured that surrogates usually met the intended parents at least once before embryo transfer and again at the birth of the child. In each of these studies, interactions with the intended parents largely informed surrogates' narratives about kinship and their relationships with the parents-to-be.

In contrast, many of the women I interviewed in Nadipur rarely if ever met their client parents. Indeed, the women often did not meet their clients until the time of birth, and sometimes not at all. Surrogates received minimal information from their doctors about the clients apart from their names and country of origin, perhaps. Within this context, how do surrogate mothers conceive of their relationships with the commissioning parents, the clients for whom they are laboring to produce a child? How do surrogates relate to the fetus during pregnancy? Postpregnancy, how do they view their relationship with the child born of their labor? In addressing these questions, I begin by elucidating how doctors articulate their own role in transnational surrogacy arrangements and how they influence the ways in which surrogates conceive of their relationships with the commissioning parents as well as the fetuses they bear. All the doctors I spoke with saw themselves as the critical link between surrogates and intended parents. They typically used this position to privilege the desires and perspectives of the commissioning parents, while disparaging the intentions and viewpoints of the surrogate mothers. In so doing they demonstrated a hierarchical approach toward their management of these relationships, racializing Indian surrogate mothers as Other and unequivocally inferior to Western intended parents. I frame these particular racial formations as expressions of physician racism that influence surrogates' views of the intended parents as well as of the fetuses they labor to gestate and birth. In contrast to cases in which commissioning parents and surrogates developed a personal relationship, which encouraged surrogates to view the commissioning mothers as "global sisters" (Pande 2011) or as "conjoined patients" who share a "linked and sometimes merged subjectivity" (Teman 2010, 184), the surrogates in this study referred to the intended parents as their "clients." I believe this reflects the doctor's devaluation of their connection and the explicit commodification of an intimate and personal relationship. In a host of ways surrogates revealed that they viewed the commissioning parents as actors in an economic transaction rather than as cocollaborators in the creation of babies or coparticipants in alternative networks of kin.

Surrogates also expressed diverse views about their relationship with the fetus or child born through surrogacy. Some women fully accept the view that they have no claim on the children they bear, while others feel a stronger bond with the child. Still others feel deep emotional distress when separated from the child, while several women only ask why they are denied the simple request of seeing the baby after birth. Throughout their narratives, surrogates relied on the language of "rights" to describe their perspectives on their relationship with the fetus; this language stems from their roles as workers in a business transaction. Drawing on Boris and Parreñas's (2010) theorization of intimate labor and Parreñas, Thai, and Silvey's (2016) conceptualization of intimate industries, I suggest that racism and a racialized labor market governs surrogates' views of their relationship with the fetus or child, as well as with the commissioning parents.

The Commodification of Intimate Relations and the Construction of Race

As theorized by Parreñas, Thai, and Silvey (2016), intimate industries provide and produce affect, care, reproduction, and sex by means of an institutionalized system. At the heart of economies of intimate exchange is the circulation of both capital and labor; such exchanges also provoke challenges to relations considered "priceless" or "not for sale." Intimate relations, in other words, depend on acts otherwise associated with being "physically and/or emotionally close, personal, sexually intimate, private, caring or loving" (Constable 2009a, 50). Commodified intimate relations often take place on unequal terrain, with one party performing the maintenance of intimacy more than the other, and they promote the well-being of the other party. Intimate industries ultimately reflect the institutionalization of commodified intimate social relations, particularly those involving marriage, sex, child care, elder care, or in this instance, reproduction.

Transnational surrogacy represents a prime example of an intimate industry, as the commodification of pregnancy and childbirth has become increasingly institutionalized at the global level. Within the systematization of the intimate labor involved in transnational surrogacy, the global market and bureaucratic rules and regulations mediate a wide set of social relations. A broad range of actors and institutions make possible the commodified labor inherent in transnational surrogacy, including social workers, family, and immigration lawyers; medical specialists, genetic counselors, embryologists, and gynecologists; travel agencies that coordinate global travel; sperm and egg banks; consulates that issue travel documents such as passports and visas; and surrogacy agencies that recruit and tend to surrogate mothers.

Within this context, questions regarding the intersection of markets and intimacy are central. Sociologist Arlie Hochschild has critiqued the commodity exchanges increasingly embedded in the intimate spheres of everyday life, such as child care, mate selection, and family making through commercial surrogacy. Throughout her works lamenting the intrusion of commodity exchange in intimate relations, Hochschild privileges the gift mode of exchange. In *The Managed Heart: Commercialization of Human Feeling* (1983) she contends that the exchange of emotions guides nonmarket social life; gift exchange principles govern these exchanges. In contrast, the commodification of emotions renders these interactions inauthentic; that is, once interaction moves from the socially driven gift exchange economy into the impersonal market, actors no longer assume the ability to freely negotiate the terms and kinds of exchange. Yet other scholars, in particular Viviana Zelizer, suggest that intimacy and economic transactions "do not stand at two opposing corners like hostile pugilists" (Zelizer 2010, 167). Rather, people combine intimate relations and economic transactions in unpredictable ways; in other words, the two are interconnected and create, define, sustain, and challenge one another. While previous studies of surrogacy have shown how actors work to separate economy from intimacy, in this chapter I show how the two are intertwined.

Central to this intersection of economy and intimacy are processes of racialization that contribute to the formation of a "racialized labor market." This market emerges from a longer history of racialized (and racist) discourses about the connections between labor, technology, and Asia and Asians. As Lee and Wong (2003) discuss, these discourses racialize Asians in particular ways, representing Asians as possessing a tense relationship with technology; they are either "nimble-fingered" female workers employed in computer factories or "geeks" writing code. Similarly, as I have discussed earlier, the dominant discourses portray Indian surrogates either as objects to be rescued or as workers simply doing a job for remuneration. Yet located within a global political economy that is stratified by race as well as gender and national location, these discourses racialize Indian surrogates on the basis of their participation in this intimate industry. This chapter investigates the role of Indian doctors in perpetuating racialized discourses about Indian surrogates, solidifying surrogates' unequal positions at the bottom of the labor market hierarchy.

However, in focusing on the role of doctors in maintaining racist discourses, I do not wish to argue that individual doctors are the cause of racialization within transnational surrogacy arrangements. Indeed, ridding the medical establishment of bad actors would not eradicate the broader structures that produce the racist and racial formations embedded in transnational surrogacy. The individual racialization of physicians occurs concurrently with broader institutional structures of racism that are responsible for patterns of inequality that empower the expansion of the global surrogacy industry.

At the same time, in demonstrating how Indian physicians racialize surrogates I do not claim that doctors and surrogates represent distinct racial groups, nor do I argue that caste or religion are identical to race in the context of contemporary India. Yet while caste, race, and religion cannot be equated, scholars have examined how these concepts are socially constructed in similar ways. Das (2014), for instance, examines the ways in which Indians essentialize and racialize caste groups on the basis of perceived immutable, inheritable, and purported biological differences, with upper-caste individuals perceived as fair and lower-caste individuals perceived as dark in spite of the existence of dark-skinned members of upper castes and light-skinned members of lower castes.

Oommen (2005) points out the implicit association between fair complexion and enlightenment. This logic reflects persistent (if inaccurate) beliefs in race as a biological construct (Omi and Winant 1986).

The salience of class, caste, and religious identities remains although it does not map neatly onto my respondents' social identities. Nor do these identities alone explain the interactions I observed. But, as I describe below, underlying ideologies of racism and caste-based discrimination intersect to create new racial formations which attach certain kinds of racial meanings to categories of surrogates, clients, and egg donors. I suggest that doctors racialize surrogates in ways that essentialize their social and biological suitability as surrogates but also their capacity for deceit and blackmail, representing them as individuals appropriate to their task but also not completely trustworthy.

The Logic of Reproductive Hierarchies: Physician Perspectives

Indian doctors' primary role in transnational surrogacy goes far beyond the function of providing medical treatment, advice, and care to surrogates and newborns. Indeed, in practice and in interviews, doctors seemed to focus very little on the medical aspects of surrogacy. Rather, they seemed preoccupied by the social and business aspects of the industry. In interviews many wondered aloud about improving efficiency and client-doctor and client-surrogate relations, and they prioritized their role as facilitators at the heart of social and business transactions. Dr. Verma exemplified this when she explained, "It's like they [surrogate mothers] are adopted by me. They travel in my car, they get everything for those ten months and then after ten months when they come and say goodbye, I think they really feel very sad." Another doctor concurred, as she described surrogates' postsurrogacy relationship with the clinic: "It's like there is this umbilical cord still attached to us; they usually call at least once a month wanting to come back and work for us." These doctors' views of their relationships with surrogates appeared to delete the existence of the commissioning parents, a predictable effect of doctors' policies of prohibiting contact between surrogates and clients.

While Dr. Verma, in giving herself the responsibility of serving as "adopted mother," at least implied she should keep the surrogates happy, Dr. Singh seemed uninterested in the happiness of surrogates. Rather, like many of the doctors I interviewed, she emphasized how anxiety-provoking the surrogacy process could be for clients and claimed she was willing to do whatever was necessary to keep them calm, happy, and well informed about every detail of the pregnancy. Ruminating on what might happen if she lost communication with the intended parents, Dr. Singh stated:

> If you stop that continuous communication, those emails saying, "Everything's okay; these are your scans. These are your videos," etc.—there's obviously going to be anxiety. . . . So I think the most important part of the surrogacy program is staying in touch with clients. It's not getting [the surrogates] pregnant because that's, you know, you've got the best uterus there—it's not an *achievement* to get them pregnant. The achievement is to keep [the clients] happy, to keep them anxiety-free through those nine months of pregnancy. To think about the amount of malaria in the city and to wonder, "Does my surrogate have malaria? Is there a water problem; could she get typhoid?" These are the things that I think of. You have to put yourself in their place and say, "What if I had a surrogate in India [while I was half a world away]?" I would just die of anxiety. I wouldn't be able to deal with it. Just thinking about it, I'd probably send them five liters of Bisleri [brand of bottled water] every day just to make sure she's drinking that water. [emphasis in the original]

Dr. Singh explicitly identified with the prospective parents in expressing her sympathy for their plight. Because she and her Western clients shared similar socioeconomic class positions she could easily imagine their anxiety. Dr. Singh constructed the population of surrogates as subject to risks unfamiliar to the Euro-American clients or the upper-class Indian doctors who treated them, marking the surrogate population as fundamentally dissimilar. She believed she and her clients would voice the same concerns about environmental and geographical influences on the poor women's access to clean water and exposure to malaria, risks that implicated the surrogates' caste and socioeconomic status. Many of Dr. Singh's surrogates came from one of the most socially disadvantaged groups in India, Dalits. As a scheduled caste, Dalits have historically been segregated and denied access to education and public places such as temples, drinking water wells, and restaurants. The research bears out Dr. Singh's implication that they have poorer health outcomes than those who belong to upper castes (Subramanian et al. 2008). Caste bear; connotations and carries with it a colonial history in which Indian historically conflated caste and race; Dr. Singh's concerns around surrogates' health were also racialized (Oommen 2002).

Explanations of communal conflict in India frequently overemphasize the importance of religion, secularism, or antisecularism and therefore obscure the importance of race and structural factors, as Dr. Singh's remarks highlight (Baber 2004). As Chakrabarty has argued, Indian society dismisses racism as the affliction of white people, ignoring that Indians can treat one another in racist ways (1994, 145). The Indian doctors I spoke with and heard about from surrogates and commissioning parents treated Indian surrogates in ways that reflect specific patterns that resemble racial conflicts in other social contexts.

Thus, aspects of caste discrimination can illustrate patterns that reflect racism in other parts of the world. Indeed, Indian scholars have argued that communal identities have in fact been racialized, so that caste and religious discrimination function as racism within India (Baber 2004; Das 2014; Oommen 2002). For example, caste discrimination manifests in residential segregation, such as the persistent residential segregation of "untouchables" in Indian villages. As Gyanendra Pandey (1993) points out, upper-caste Hindus claim the right to rule and live in comfort and security as an inherited right, and consider the subordination of lower-caste Hindus as appropriate to their birth. Religion, class, nation, and caste function as markers of racialized identities in India; when Indian surrogates provide services to Euro-American clients, these markers have weight.

Dr. Singh's remark that surrogates provide "the best uterus there [is]," likewise links lower-caste Indian women to their biological reproductive capacities, essentializing poor Indian women's suitability for pregnancy and racializing the population of Indian surrogates as biologically more appropriate for surrogacy work than their upper-caste counterparts. It also highlights the perceived fecundity of lower-class Indian women, a belief that extends back to early twentieth-century antinatalist debates in India in which the Indian elite believed that the modern Indian state needed to restrain the perceived excessive fertility of subaltern women, especially lower-class, lower-caste, and Muslim women (Jolly and Ram 2001). Moreover, it reduces the Indian surrogate to her womb, reflecting

Cooper and Waldby's (2014) insight that reproductive technologies fragment women's bodies into parts and processes in order to commodify the reproductive part desired in a particular transaction.

Dr. Singh's clinic interfaced directly with surrogates just as it did with commissioning parents. Yet she described her interactions with surrogates in far less sympathetic terms:

> They might call me and say, "You know, my back is hurting." I say, "You just went to the doctor this afternoon. Why didn't you tell her?" "No, but we know only you." They will call you up for the *ridiculous stuff* that happens to them. They need that one person who they can just pick up the phone and complain to. There are some who nag you every single day. [emphasis in the original]

Unlike Dr. Verma, who framed surrogates' emotional attachment in at least somewhat positive terms, Dr. Singh viewed surrogates' concerns as insignificant and "ridiculous."

Dr. Singh's biases became even more apparent when she discussed the clinic's management of the surrogates and the problems of maintaining communication with them. She believed these problems might derail her former employer, Origins:

> Dr. Jain has decided to look after the program herself, and that actually kind of worries me because she doesn't have the time for this and she needs a subordinate who could carry out the day-to-day [tasks] with surrogates and be on-call on her cell phone to tell them what's happening to them. And once you lose the rapport with the surrogate and you lose the rapport with the client, the link is lost. How does one keep both of them happy? That one person *has* to be there. [emphasis in the original]

The subordinate Dr. Singh mentioned fit into a pyramid-like structure that many critics of surrogacy generally denounce, claiming that a system that supports caretakers, agents, and brokers intrinsically exploits both the surrogates who provide the core labor and the clients who must fund all the parties involved. But Dr. Singh argued that the difficulty of communicating with surrogates and intended parents required that Dr. Jain have a "subordinate" to help her. This subordinate, often a nurse, social worker, or agent, controls much of the dissemination of information to surrogates. Indeed, many surrogates described how processes of consent and information about various medical procedures came not from the doctor but from the agent who introduced them to the clinic. In all these interactions, doctors and their subordinates communicate directly with the surrogate and the client. Facilitating personal relationships between surrogate and client, however, seems unnecessary for many doctors.

Dr. Singh herself employed a subordinate at her new clinic, a former surrogate who fielded surrogates' concerns, escorted them to their medical appointments, and attended to their day-to-day needs. But Dr. Singh expressed the doubt that she would be able to delegate effectively:

> After a while you kind of stop taking their phone calls. . . . I'm trying to work the system so that there is another one appointed, someone else who is going to look after them, but then the fear is that the surrogates will still want to call me. That much I know. Because for them, you know, their mind doesn't come on time.

This expression "their mind doesn't come on time" suggested that surrogates are uneducated and stubborn. Dr. Singh lamented the difficulty of convincing surrogates not to call her about delays in payment, even though the clinic's office staff handled payments. She also complained that they would call her about problems with surrogate housing, saying that her response to hearing that the gas was out was to wonder, "What do you want me to do, come and cook?" Had she respected the surrogates more she might have recognized that they rightly saw her economic leverage in the management of housing, as the clinic had a relationship with surrogate housing, as well as her managerial position in relation to the office. But instead she focused on the fact that her efforts to discourage these calls by, for example, never distributing pay at the clinic itself, had been unsuccessful. She viewed the surrogates' concerns as irritating inconveniences and cast them as obstinate, oblivious, and irrational, even though access to cooking gas and payment as promised may well have been serious issues for them. Under the assumption that surrogates' social and health concerns were easily separable, concerns around surrogates' health and welfare were well founded only when clients articulated them as worries in relation to fetal health.

Dr. Singh in fact expressed some guilt for her treatment of the surrogates and used this guilt to further justify her desire for a subordinate who would handle the surrogates:

> So there are days when you are patient and you are good with them and then there are days when you lose it, when you completely lose it. And you feel really bad about yelling at them sometimes, and you know, my husband gets shocked—he asks, "Who are you talking to like that?" But there is a certain level of stubbornness in *that class of people.* You know, it's hard to make them understand. They won't understand because literacy is hardly here and they just don't want to understand anyone else's problem. They say, "You do something about it." So that's something that's really bothering me right now. Who is going to be that next person who will be the point of contact, because once the IVF flow does increase, I don't see myself doing this for very long. [emphasis in the original]

Dr. Singh's characterization of surrogates as "that class of people" who were illiterate reveals the class-imbued nature of her feelings about surrogates. In fact my observations suggest that the educational levels of Indian women who enlist in surrogacy vary widely. I interviewed women who had low levels of educational attainment, with a substantial number completing only a primary school education; I also interviewed many women who had completed high school and several who had completed college. For Dr. Singh the figure of the uneducated surrogate stood in for the entire surrogate population, erasing their diversity and subjectivity.

The description of surrogates as "*that class of people*" clearly emphasized Dr. Singh's identity as an upper-class doctor as well. Dr. Singh relied on perceptions of insurmountable difference across class, caste, and national lines in order to justify her treatment of the surrogates. Consequently, when class and caste are used to signify profound Otherness, it becomes clear that such beliefs and stereotypes about the ways in which the population of surrogates "just are" can be just as pernicious and racist as racism.

When I asked Dr. Singh to say more about the problems surrogates encountered, she stated:

> Most of the problems that we're facing are social and they've got nothing to do with medicine. They've got nothing to do with IVF. . . . For ex-

ample, refusing to shift into the housing. They say their children are going to school, so it's too far. That's becoming a nuisance now, actually. Despite speaking with them before the transfer, making sure they will shift, there's this attitude that suddenly comes in once they're pregnant. They don't want to move now. This just happened to me two weeks ago. They already signed the documents and I told them they've got to move now. They're supposed to shift with their families, so the husband calls me up threatening me, saying, "But the whole thing was in English. We didn't understand it." I said, "But I spoke to you in Hindi. Didn't you understand that?" So the point is, yeah, they'll come around eventually. But the amount of stress that you go through and the way you need to speak to them, it's not fun. You don't feel good about it [laughing a little]. You don't feel good about the sternness that comes into your voice. And the threat that you have to put forth, saying, "You know, you do this, you don't move in and I'm going to have to call the police because you signed the agreement."

Here again Dr. Singh revealed that her antagonistic treatment of the surrogates caused her discomfort, but she emphasized that the surrogates rarely had physical problems during pregnancy. Her comments reflect a power dynamic in which doctors always have the upper hand, exercising the power to tell the surrogate what to do and even to threaten legal action if they do not obey. The surrogates had no input into decisions regarding their housing, treatment, or family lives. Indeed, Dr. Singh dismissed the importance of the surrogate's child's education—a concern she would presumably have validated if an upper-caste person had expressed it—and focused on the stress she herself experienced in these interactions, which must pale in comparison to that of a family that must uproot itself and leave a school or be separated. SUR. PROB!

Throughout our interview Dr. Singh's phone rang constantly, supporting her claim that surrogates contacted her frequently. She ignored the first two calls but spoke to a surrogate on the third. Hanging up after a brief conversation in Hindi, she turned to me and said in exasperation:

Here is the kind of trash you face. . . . The surrogate's sister is calling me up and she's been calling me since morning. She says this lady's 31, 32 weeks pregnant now and she's got twins and she's been admitted since the past ten days, because she was threatening to go into labor [and the hospital was trying to stop it]. . . . And the sister calls up and says, "Get the babies out." It's very troublesome. But see, this attitude that, you know, how can you think about delivering prematurely? Would you have done it if it were your own? Then, the only language that works with them is, "Okay, we'll get the babies out right now. You'll only take just half the money."

When I asked how surrogates handled this threat—which might well constitute a breach of contract—Dr. Singh said that they always backed down when she made it. She told me,

I have no other way of handling them. It's kind of sad that they even think that way. And that's why I think when I started off I think I got conned into so many things because I just trusted them. And now I'm seeing the other side of it and you get wiser every time. You start losing respect. You know, at some point in time, you cannot treat all of them the same way. Because one out of maybe fifty is going to be genuine and actually cares about the pregnancy, etc. The remaining forty-nine, it's a business transaction, that's about it.

Dr. Singh's description of the surrogate's sister's concerns as "trash" revealed her utter lack of concern for the surrogate's health; her sole concern was ensuring the health of the babies. Indeed, Dr. Singh implied that she occupied herself primarily with the health of the fetuses because the surrogates themselves held their pregnancies in such low regard. Such characterizations rely on binaries in which the surrogate will concern herself with either the child or her payment, as if the two were mutually exclusive.

Dr. Singh construction of surrogates as untrustworthy, scheming figures undeserving of her respect mirrors racialized constructions of the "welfare queen" and the "wily patient" in Khiara Bridges's (2011) study of pregnancy as a site of racialization in a New York City public hospital. Bridges demonstrates how medical providers discursively produce and implicitly racialize as black the figure of the "wily patient" and the "welfare queen." She simultaneously calls attention to the ways in which these figures represent the racialization of persistent archetypes—in the case of the welfare queen, the archetype of undeservingness. I suggest that participants in the transnational surrogacy industry racialize surrogates as the archetype of the scheming, deviant, low-caste woman (see Gupta 2008). By virtue of the very fact that she enlisted in commercial surrogacy in order to earn money, the presumed low-class, low-caste surrogate emerges as an uneducated, irrational figure, morally suspect and not to be trusted. Indeed, Dr. Singh positioned herself as a victim of surrogates who took advantage of her, just as a welfare queen might take advantage of the government. Such racialized constructions of surrogate mothers set the stage for doctors' justifications for the ways in which they structure client-surrogate relationships.

Organizing Client-Surrogate Relationships

Most doctors I spoke with agreed with Dr. Singh that meetings between surrogates and clients could encourage "blackmail." Doctors structure relations between clients and surrogates to the advantage of commissioning clients as they see fit. As Dr. Doshi, an infertility specialist based in Mumbai, explained, "We discourage communication between surrogates and clients. For them, it is basically an emotional issue; but I think it is the womb that is important. It is not necessary to see where the person stays, how the person looks. By looking at a person, if we think she's not good, we will form an opinion; but if her uterus is good—she can carry a pregnancy. And surrogates will start demanding extra money after knowing it is a foreign couple. They may say, 'I'm in pain; I will abort the child. I need Rs. 50,000.' Who will pay? It has happened with others." Yet, while surrogates told me that they wished to know more about their clients, Dr. Verma claimed to speak for them, saying, "The surrogate doesn't want anybody to be in touch or turning up at her door. So they're not interested, you know." Dr. Singh agreed, though she admitted, "I'm not saying that they're not human and wouldn't probably want to meet. [Surrogates] would probably want to know who's finally taking the baby back."

Dr. Verma practiced in Delhi and had a large foreign clientele. She explained her policy regarding contact between clients and surrogates as follows:

My policy is that I don't allow any gifts and they have just one basic meeting before the embryo transfer. After that, I don't encourage any person-to-person contact at all. After the baby is born, I tell the intended parents:

"You can gift her your house, you can gift her your entire bank balance. That is up to you; but wait until the baby is handed over, until your contract is over." I set it up this way because I don't want to even have a suggestion or a hint of any sort of problem. They are very different culturally, the two sides. And they don't understand what the other person is trying to say. They may misperceive each other's actions. . . . And really, you know, what is there to talk about? I mean, at the end of the day, once the baby's handed over, it's not like they are going to be in touch.

Other researchers found that surrogates and parents in other parts of the world expected to stay in contact even after the birth of the child, even though, as in Dr. Verma's practice, the surrogates had no genetic link to the child (Teman 2010). But Dr. Verma believed her clients and their Indian surrogates would have no desire to keep in touch. She tied this to the cultural gulf between the two parties. Here, "culture" stands in for "race," in that "culture is understood to be an indicator of difference that is both immutable and impossible to negotiate" (Bridges 2011, 136). Indeed, Dr. Verma emphasized differences in phenotype and skin color to illustrate why surrogates held no claim on or kin relationship to the baby: "I tell the surrogates, 'The baby doesn't look like you and the baby is not yours.' So they understand."

Dr. Singh also suggested that any help extended by clients to surrogates should follow the handing over of the baby:

I think to be manipulated by emotions [by surrogates] at that point in time is not fair. You can help the surrogate out in so many ways later. But it's just that when the demand starts coming from the other end, that's what starts annoying me. You know, they say, "Have they left anything for me? They haven't met me."

For doctors, the construction of surrogates as largely ignorant and uneducated because of their lower-class status exists alongside a competing, contradictory view of the surrogate population as shrewd manipulators of intended parents, with financial gain being the sole motive.

The ways in which doctors constructed surrogates and explained their policies of restricting contact influenced the intended parents. For instance, the Canadian Turkish couple Sharon and Ahmet were undergoing their first attempt at surrogacy in India after a long history of infertility and multiple attempts at altruistic surrogacy in their home country. Sharon explained what she viewed as the primary differences between surrogacy in Canada and India.

> Here, the surrogates, they don't want any connections. It's not that we mind if she wants a picture or something, but we don't want any emotional bonding. It seemed like a lot of the ladies in Canada want you to live next to them, or they want you to have some sort of relationship. That's their option, right, if that's what they're looking for. But we feel content this way [in India]; there's no need to be getting into each other's lives, and it seems like that's how a lot of ladies here prefer it.

While Sharon had not yet met or spoken with a surrogate, clearly doctors' views about the surrogates influence intended parents. Moreover, Sharon reflected on the fact that the sheer geographical and cultural distance between the surrogates and intended parents made surrogacy in India so attractive to her. Rather than pursue surrogacy in Canada, where surrogates would expect some level of involvement with the commissioning parents, Sharon saw the vast cultural and geographical distance between herself and the Indian surrogate as an opportunity to engage in surrogacy without the hassle of emotional connection. As Lisa Ikemoto (2009) argues, it is the very racial, cultural, and economic differences—a form of "racial distancing"—that makes gestational surrogacy palatable to commissioning clients.

When Dr. Singh said, "Getting them pregnant is the easier part. It's the nine months which is difficult," she clearly viewed the challenges embedded in transnational surrogacy as social rather than medical. Yet data indicate that assisted reproductive technologies are rife with low success rates; it's just that the social problems pose the hardest challenge to doctors. I have argued that doctors' articulations of surrogates' "social problems" are a form of racialization that positions surrogates as a racialized group, characterized by low education, low income, and low caste status. Moreover, their participation in the surrogacy industry marks the women as Other to the clients who hire them, and doctors encourage this understanding by constructing surrogates as manipulative figures with little regard for the fetuses they carry. I argue that these racialized constructions of surrogates play a significant role in the way surrogates themselves understand their relationships with intended parents. Yet as I describe below, these conceptions of kinship and relatedness are not clear-cut and surrogates develop creative strategies for constructing their own notions of relatedness.

On Kinship and Relatedness: Surrogates' Views

By interviewing women over the course of their pregnancies and several years postpregnancy, I noticed shifts in opinions over time as well as the diversity of women's experiences with surrogacy. Their feelings about the intended parents ranged from disinterest to resentment.

Surrogates' Disinterest

Several surrogates I interviewed indicated that they had little use for detailed information about their clients, just as the doctors had described. I first met Parvati when she became pregnant as a surrogate for a foreign couple in 2010. Early in her pregnancy I asked about her interest in the couple for whom she had become pregnant. Parvati replied:

> What will I do with any knowledge about them? It will be of no use to me. I have seen them here [briefly, at the time of the embryo transfer] but they never talked to me except for some greetings and questions regarding my health, and I don't think they'll talk to me again. Often they talk with the doctor only.

Parvati saw the clients as having little interest in speaking with her and felt no interest in disrupting this. Yet she also mentioned that when she met the couple, the doctor "didn't allow" her to have "a chat with them." Thus while Parvati expressed indifference about her relationship with the clients, she also implicitly held the doctor responsible for her lack of any connection with them, suggesting that she might have been open to a relationship with the intended parents if the doctor had allowed it.

Surrogate Hena responded similarly when I asked about her clients. At the time of our first interview, Hena had just undergone embryo transfer. While she saw the same doctor as Parvati, Hena had not met her clients and knew very little about them. When I asked if she'd like to know them or to meet the clients, she responded:

> What is the purpose in meeting them? There is no reason for which I should meet them anyway. I'm a surrogate and it doesn't matter to me who is going to take the baby. What I've got to do is deliver the baby, take the payment, and go. The only strange feeling I do have about the process is that I'm going to give the child away after keeping it in me for nine months.

When asked if she knew where her clients were from, Hena replied, "I don't know at all." Seated next to Hena was her friend Ashima, who was also in the same stage of the process. Ashima concurred: "Honestly speaking, I don't feel like meeting them. I also feel like Hena; that is the fact." These interactions played out in the ways that the doctors anticipated; doctors who work to create and maintain a distance between the two parties hope that the surrogates will view their role as Hena, Ashima, and Parvati did. This reinforces doctors' views that a surrogate who wishes to connect with the intended parents is solely concerned with remuneration.

In a desire compatible with the idea that surrogates have little interest in the clients' point of view, some surrogates felt that clients should show them respect, and that they typically failed to do so. Antara, who was a former surrogate as well as an agent, argued that surrogacy actually worked better with couples from abroad; Indian couples tended to meddle in surrogates' lives too much. Yet she felt that an ideal relationship would be one of respect:

> In one case, Anu's case, the client never showed the courtesy of greeting us or giving good wishes to her after she delivered twins for them and went through cesarean. They just paid their amount and took the kids away. Surrogates really feel bad after being treated in this way. They are not asking you for something extra and they are also aware that you are the original parents of the kids. There is no harm in showing some humanity but they didn't even look at her once.

Antara's comment that surrogates "are not asking for something extra" contradicts doctors' views that surrogates are indifferent to the treatment of intended parents and will attempt to extort money from the clients if given the opportunity. She described acknowledgment from clients for the work they had completed as a courtesy and its omission as a lack of respect. Many surrogate mothers I spoke with described such markers of disrespect as troubling.

Former surrogate Padma, for example, told me that when she was recovering from her cesarean section:

> They did not even come to see me. They didn't even come to look at me. And from the beginning until the birth of the daughter, we did not meet at all. They came only once into the room, talked to the doctor, and then just left. They did not ask about how I am. They should have just asked. Otherwise what is there to give and take?

Padma described a sense of abandonment and disrespect. When Padma stated, "what is there to give and take?" she challenged the idea that surrogacy is unquestionably a mutually beneficial arrangement between surrogates and clients; rather, the parents' lack of respect for Padma and her labor implied an unequal relationship that left her feeling let down.

Although Hena professed not to care whether she had any contact with the intended parents, she faulted the doctors directly for the distance:

> The main thing is, [the doctors] do not allow us to meet clients personally, or talk to them in person. If there is a good client who pays well, they will not allow the patients [surrogates] to meet them. [The doctors] tell us to lie to them, they tell us to say "yes" to any questions about whether we are eating well, etc.

Hena noted that the doctor she worked with, Dr. Desai, usually prohibited surrogates from meeting high-paying foreign clients. Her description of being instructed to lie contrasts with the charge that surrogates were conniving and would seek to extort money from clients.

In the context of a relationship doctors encouraged them to view as purely transactional, surrogates argued that the lack of communication doctors imposed on them placed them in an unequal position. While Hena had disparaged the idea of needing an emotional connection with the client, she felt that she should have been able to discuss business with the couple directly:

> The doctor should allow us to meet the other party. Whatever is done, should be done in person. I mean, when payment is to be discussed, the clients should speak with us directly. If we agree, we will do it; if we don't agree, we won't do it. But there should not be so much distance.

Many women agreed with Hena, describing their inability to discuss the economic terms of their relationship directly with the clients as extremely frustrating.

Salma, a former surrogate, did not distinguish between business and emotional reasons to meet with clients. She said, "I mean, you don't need to meet very frequently, but while doing ET [embryo transfer], at least once they should meet you. If your own wife was pregnant, would you have kept her so far away from you?" Salma was the only surrogate who described herself to me as analogous to a spouse in the transaction. In this she articulated that she was more than a "womb for rent" and that she deserved the respect a husband pays a wife when she's pregnant.

This sense of playing a familial role did not conflict with the sense of being entitled to fair compensation. She said:

> See, if we go and ask somebody for a rupee, nobody will give. So this is our earning from the hard work. We have a right to demand this from them. Right? When we feel that our compensation is less, then we can tell you that this amount is less; give us more. This is our hard earned money. We cannot ask for this from others.

When Salma said that if she asked, "nobody will give," she acknowledged the difference between begging for money and working for it. She believed surrogates have the right to demand money in exchange for their hard work and to negotiate their payments directly with the consumers hiring them for their reproductive labor. While doctors framed the surrogates' demands for money in terms of blackmail, Salma referred to the surrogate's right to negotiate her own financial compensation.

Salma also distinguished the work of surrogacy from "dirty work," that is, prostitution: "If a woman does a dirty job, then her respect is gone and people also talk bad about her. So then, it is better to do this work. We do a holy work for god. We bring a baby into this world." Salma said this in the context of a group discussion with a dozen surrogates, former surrogates, agents, and egg donors. Hearing her statement, the other women in the room spontaneously applauded, the only time this happened in the course of my fieldwork.

The results of doctors' racialization of women as simultaneously uneducated and manipulative, ignorant and shrewd, and ultimately too untrustworthy to be allowed to communicate with the clients directly encouraged the surrogates to view their relationships with would-be parents in primarily transactional terms. I argue that if doctors approached these relationships differently, the women would not consistently refer to commissioning parents as "clients" and they would not feel that the process deprived them of their dignity or financial agency. Yet many surrogates' narratives belied doctors' claims that surrogates treated their role as transactional. Indeed, their comments about their connection to the fetuses they carried reveal the wide-ranging effects of the racial formations that essentialize them.

On Bonding with the Fetus

Conversations among women indicated that there was often disagreement about the effect of surrogacy on women's feelings toward the baby. Salma and Hena, for instance, revealed their disparate opinions in the following conversation:

SALMA: When the baby is conceived, then we know clearly that it is not our baby, so we do not let the attachment grow. What we only do is eat and drink so that the baby is healthy.

HENA: But I had my attachment with the baby. I am still attached with the baby. Last month was her birthday. I still sit and cry.

S: Yes, you feel like crying. But when you give, you think it is somebody else's and not ours. If it is ours, then of course we do let attachment grow.

H: But I had a daughter [via surrogacy]. And now I feel that, look, my daughter was born. I do not have a daughter [with me] now, but I delivered one.

Both women understood that clients and doctors expected them to have no emotional attachment to the baby. Yet Hena expressed her pain upon giving away "her daughter." Parvati said that following the birth of the twin girls she had carried, "I felt bad. The clients did not give anything. They didn't give me any photos of my daughters. They didn't give phone numbers. They did not even show them to me." Here, while Parvati did not express any interest in knowing the clients, she felt connected to the twins, referring to them as "my daughters," contradicting doctors' assertions that these were not "their" children. Similarly, Mansi said, "But [surrogacy] is not a thing like a dream. It is not only of a day; it is a thing of nine months. What is the difference between our child and their child?" Parvati's sadness at not even receiving a phone number indicates that the surrogates want to remain in contact with the clients because of the children they carried, belying doctors' claims that surrogates have no desire to stay in touch once the contract is completed. Such remarks illustrate the ways in which surrogates navigate the relationships forged through commercial surrogacy, relations that do not always adhere to dominant medical models of kinship and relatedness.

Antara, on the other hand, did not view the child she had birthed through surrogacy as one of her "own." Reflecting on the question of how she would react, at some point in the future, to reconnecting with the child to which she gave birth, she replied, "We may feel nice and treat him nicely, but we'll not feel as lovingly as we feel for our children. It will be like any other relative visiting us on some day." Here, although Antara did not "kin" the child as one of her own, she acknowledged that the child may be considered family, "like any other relative" she might encounter.

Yet during another interview Antara disparaged the idea that surrogacy is solely a financial arrangement: "We grow the child like our own for nine months inside us. Money does not matter always. We have done something for the child as well. Is it only for money? The need was from both sides, but we have attached to it too. We feel very sad while giving it away." She admitted that she remembered the birthday of the baby she had relinquished, and that she had tried to call the family—who were Indian and lived in north India—to wish the child a happy birthday, but could not reach anyone: "I called him. But I could not reach him. They change their numbers. But you still remember." Yamini interjected,

"Some people do change their numbers even after they have given it to us." This behavior, of deliberately refusing to maintain a line of contact with the surrogates, contrasts sharply with that of parents in other studies of surrogacy.

A later interview with both Antara and Yamini revealed another change. When I asked them how they felt when handing the baby over, they replied:

> ANTARA: Nothing. We don't have any feeling for the child as we are aware that the child is not our own.
>
> YAMINI: They take it before we can see it after delivering it. What could anyone feel if she is not even allowed to see the baby?"
>
> A: No, in my case the baby was with me for the next three days. But still I didn't feel anything for it. But the system of not allowing surrogates to see the babies is right because they might feel something for the baby, which is risky. Kali's sister-in-law delivered a girl as a surrogate and the baby was taken away, but she was crying like anything to get a glimpse of it. She was telling everybody that the baby was hers only. Then they took a photograph of the baby and gave it to her to calm her down.

While Antara praised the practice of separating babies from surrogates, she acknowledged that women feel an attachment. Antara went on to explain that seeing the photograph probably helped Kali's sister-in-law, but said that the doctors later revised their policies to avoid such problems. Such policies influenced Swati's feelings about the children she had birthed: "No, I don't feel anything toward the children. I wanted to see my kids but the doctors did not allow me to see them at all. Once I knew that they were not allowing me even to see, then I said, ok, that's it, end of story. And when we know that the babies are not ours, then why should we insist on seeing them now?" Swati's comments reflect the contradictory ways in which women often understood their relationships to the babies: they were simultaneously "my kids" and "not ours." Following the doctors' policies, however, Swati lost any desire to even see the babies following birth.

In a pattern I believe reflects a desire to distinguish the emotional effects of a pregnancy that produced their genetic child from one produced through surrogacy, some women argued that the physical changes surrogates experience during pregnancy are different from those experienced during their previous pregnancies. During a visit to Antara's home at which several women were present—all surrogates in varying stages of pregnancy—one surrogate's husband was present and wanted to hear more about the physical changes in their pregnancies and how these might be different from their previous pregnancies. Yamini and Antara discussed it as follows:

> YAMINI: I don't think that the process will bring any changes in the surrogate because there is no relation with anybody—I mean all the physical changes that are normally observed in women after delivering a baby. Some become fat, some thin, some may become fair or dark. But in surrogacy, women don't have any physical relations. I don't think a surrogate is getting the same things happening to her as with a normal woman after delivery because there is no physical relation with anybody.
>
> ANTARA: No, it is the same. There is no difference between these two deliveries.
>
> Y: Most importantly we don't feel anything at the time of giving the baby to the couple because we are not at all attached to it.

Yamini suggested that pregnancy caused by sexual intercourse would change a woman's body in ways that ART would not, ignoring Antara's disagreement (and scientific logic). She explicitly related this distinction to emotional distance, creating a link between the physical and psychological changes in "normal" versus surrogate pregnancies.

Many women described themselves with more consistency than Antara and Yamini as indifferent to the babies they gestated and birthed. The women often relied on this language of "rights" and "claims." Samita explained, "There is no right of me on this baby," while Paramita concurred, "Yes, I do not have any right to this baby; this baby does not belong to me." In a twist on the ubiquitous "wombs-for-rent" trope, Anusha described the child as a house that is rented, not to be claimed as the surrogate's own: "Surrogates do not have any right to claim anything on the babies. It is like somebody taking a house on rent and claiming it as his own." They referenced their explicit renunciation of any rights.

The women clearly held wide-ranging views on their relationship with the fetus or child born through surrogacy. Yet while they viewed the commissioning parents strictly as "clients," highlighting the transactional basis of their relationship, they described a more ambivalent relationship with the fetus. While many women fully accepted the contractual terms that denied surrogates any right to claim the baby, others grew attached to the babies. In both cases, the surrogates' notions of kinship and relatedness within the families created by surrogacy stemmed from their understanding of rights and labor. On the one hand, their notions of kinship coincided with the rights outlined in the contract; the women were not to bond with or lay claim to children who were not "theirs." On the other, the women articulated their desire to know or see their child in terms of rights—rights to which they were entitled as reproductive laborers.

In this chapter I have explored the ways in which ideologies of racism and caste-based discrimination contribute to new racial formations in the context of transnational surrogacy. As doctors construct their clients and the population of surrogates in particular ways, they develop racial reproductive imaginaries through which they justify their treatment of surrogates and clients. Surrogates described this treatment as making it impossible to communicate or negotiate directly with the clients, aware that this hindered their ability to lobby on their own behalf. They perceived their inability to negotiate face-to-face as a mark of disrespect. The fact that they were also engaged in the making of families was secondary.

As I will discuss in the following chapter, physician practices of racialization have significant implications for women's medical experiences as well, as these practices produce the bodies of poor surrogate mothers as requiring and deserving of medical control, a form of "racialized medicalization."

6

Medicalized Birth and the Construction of Risk

India's rate of cesarean deliveries—15 percent in public hospitals and 28 percent in private ones (IIPS 2007)—reflects the broader increase in surgical deliveries around the world. Cesarean rates rise with socioeconomic status and educational level in India, where many poor women labor outside hospitals. However, India's flourishing commercial surrogacy industry is bringing the procedure to increasing numbers of poor women who would otherwise have no access to the private, high-tech medical care that facilitates their cesarean deliveries. The medical interventions and procedures that attend high-tech medical care expose surrogate mothers to significant physical and psychosocial risks, with cesarean sections chief among the causes.

In the previous chapter I demonstrated how transnational surrogacy relies on the work of doctors to organize and facilitate relationships between commissioning clients and Indian surrogates, arguing that doctors racialize the population of surrogates in particular ways in order to justify the lack of contact between clients and surrogates. In this chapter, I extend this analysis to examine how medical discourse and doctors' views of surrogates influence the kind of medical care they receive. How does biotechnology (and the process of biomedicalization) racialize populations into social groups requiring high-tech medicalized care? I suggest that doctors' practices produce the bodies of poor surrogate mothers as a racialized social group necessitating social and medical control, thus justifying the excessive medicalization of surrogate women's bodies. Central to this process of "racialized medicalization" is the construction of surrogates' bodies as inherently risky. Racializing this population of women helps to situate their bodies as intrinsically dangerous and in need of highly medicalized care. However, while medical discourse can powerfully racialize groups of individuals as naturally perilous, it also naturalizes societal inequalities.

Within this context, I examine the medical technologies and treatments that Indian women endure as part of the surrogacy process. Doctors' approaches to cesarean section and the ways in which surrogates understand and experience pregnancy and cesarean delivery—perhaps the most medicalized type of birth—reveal the relationship between medicalization and racialization at work in transnational surrogacy. More broadly, I take up the question of how political economies and reproductive bodies shape each other. What influences the medicalized care that surrogates receive? How does surrogacy across geographic scales solidify the global inequalities in which poor bodies labor to reproduce? In addressing these questions, I elucidate the relationship between bodily labor and commercial value, examining the intersection of bodies, technology, and economy and how medicalized practices naturalize social inequality.

This chapter interrogates the intersections of commercial surrogacy and cesarean section in order to demonstrate how surrogate mothers, doctors, and intended parents experience and actively address social inequalities and processes of racialization. My goal is to draw attention to the risks and prevalence of cesarean deliveries among surrogate mothers in India and to contextualize women's experiences of surrogacy and childbirth in order to show how gestational surrogacy and cesarean delivery are inextricably intertwined. These interrelated processes, I argue, stem from practices that racialize this group of women as inherently risky, which simultaneously erases from view the risks that surrogates themselves must bear. These processes justify the use and medicalization of Indian women's bodies for the purposes of commercial surrogacy. However, such processes are fragmented and complex, as surrogate mothers too argue that their scars merit access to economic and political rights previously denied.

Intersecting Health Risks: Cesarean Sections and Assisted Reproductive Technology

In a cesarean section, the surgeon cuts through the skin and fat of the lower abdomen, slices through the tough underlying fascia, and pulls apart the muscles of the abdominal wall. Opening the peritoneum, a thin sac that encases the abdominal and pelvic organs, the surgeon peels the bladder away from the uterus, cuts open the uterus itself, and pulls out the baby and placenta. All of this can usually be done in a minute or two; the remainder of the operation consists of suturing or stapling together the layers previously cut. (Wendland 2007, 219)

Obstetrical surgery is now a routine practice, but it was once a procedure performed only when women were near death; few women survived these early operations at the end of the nineteenth century. By the 1930s, however, advances in surgical techniques helped reduce maternal mortality to below 20 percent in the United States, and obstetricians reviewing case reports realized that the timing of the cesarean was perhaps more important than the technique (Speert 1980). Indeed, women who underwent the operation early in labor, or even prior to the onset of labor, were far less likely to die (Eastman 1932). As a result, doctors performed cesarean deliveries earlier in labor and maternal mortality dropped proportionately, so that by 1965 the U.S. rate of cesareans had risen to 4.5 percent and mortality had dropped to less than 1 percent (Jones 1976).

Abdominal surgery initially grew as a means of saving the mother's life when vaginal delivery proved too risky, but doctors soon came to view it as a means of saving a fetus in danger. Electronic fetal monitoring proliferated in the developed world in the 1960s and 1970s, as did doctors' fear of claims of negligence, which signaled a turn to defensive obstetrics. Cesarean deliveries for fetal indications soared. In the United States, the rate of cesarean delivery rose from 4.5 percent in 1965 to 22.7 percent in 1985 (Taffel, Placek, and Liss 1987). In the 1970s and 1980s feminists and consumer advocates critiqued the rapid increase (Arms 1975; Cohen and Estner 1983), attacking the U.S. obstetrical system as one in which male physicians viewed women's bodies as essentially dysfunctional (Corea 1985). As patients, insurance companies, and medical professionals voiced their concerns, obstetricians began to exercise increased caution. But while the rapid increase in surgical delivery slowed in the 1980s, rates of cesarean deliveries have been climbing since the 1990s. Since 2010 U.S. rates have hovered around 32.8 percent, with nearly 1.3 million women in the United States undergoing cesarean deliveries in 2012 (Hamilton, Martin, and Ventura 2013).[1]

The rise in cesareans is a global phenomenon, one that deserves serious attention from scholars, activists, and medical and public health professionals. In a 2007–08 WHO study of the relation between method of delivery and maternal and perinatal outcomes in nine Asian countries, researchers found that the increasing rates of cesarean delivery do not necessarily lead to improved outcomes and could be associated with harm. Within this context, the rising overall rates ranging from 20 percent in Nepal to 46 percent in China are troubling. The WHO recommends that a cesarean should be done only when there is a medical indication to improve outcomes for mother and baby (Lumbiganon et al. 2010).

While the cesarean rate in India is only 18 percent overall, rates vary widely across regions and states (Lumbiganon et al. 2010). In 2005–06, the state of Kerala reported a 30 percent rate, on par with countries with the highest cesarean rates in the world, and Chennai a 45 percent rate (Ghosh and James 2010). The proportion of cesarean deliveries in urban areas is three times as high (18 percent) as in rural areas (6 percent) (Ghosh and James 2010), and doctors have estimated the rates of cesarean surgery in India's urban areas to be as high as 50 percent, with the prevalence rising to 80 percent or more in some private hospitals (Iyer and Masand 2011).

Scholars have drawn attention to climbing cesarean rates as an issue of international public health concern. Although cesarean delivery reduces overall risk in breech presentations, it also increases the risk of severe maternal and neonatal morbidity and mortality in cephalic (head-first) presentations (Villar et al. 2007). While the risk of maternal mortality for vaginal delivery is 2.5 per 100,000, the risk for women undergoing cesarean is eight times as high, at 20 per 100,000 (Boehm and Graves 1994). Other maternal complications include severe blood loss requiring transfusion, cesarean hysterectomies, wound sepsis, and anesthetic complications, as well as later complications such as incisional hernia. Moreover, primary cesarean deliveries often lead to repeat cesareans for subsequent births, with the repeat procedure carrying even higher risks for the mother. Babies born via cesarean delivery also endure their share of risks, including iatrogenic prematurity and injury due to uterine incision and extraction (Pai et al. 1999).

These risks, coupled with those associated with ART treatment, make surrogates and the children they carry especially vulnerable to a host of health and psychosocial complications. Perhaps the single most important health effect of ART treatment for both mother and child is multiple fetal pregnancy. Researchers link ART to a thirty-fold increase in multiple pregnancies compared with the rate of spontaneous twin pregnancies (1 percent in the general white population) (ACOG 2005). Twins conceived by IVF are at significantly higher risk for prematurity and neonatal morbidity and mortality than spontaneously conceived twins (Moise et al. 1998). Researchers have noted that the use of assisted reproductive technology accounts for a disproportionate number of low birth weight and very low birth weight babies in the United States, reflecting both multiple gestations and higher rates of low birth weight among singleton infants conceived through ART (Schieve et al. 2002).

Multiple pregnancies also bring a host of obstetric risks to the mother, including pregnancy-induced hypertension, preeclampsia, gestational diabetes, and preterm delivery. These risks (along with breech or shoulder presentation of at least one of the fetuses) carry a higher likelihood of complications to the mother during labor, and are named as the primary causes for the high rates of cesarean delivery in multiple pregnancies. Thus the rising numbers of multiple pregnancies conceived via ART, along with the accompanying risks, have led to increasing rates of cesarean deliveries around the world. In Australia, for example, researchers found that half of all women who conceived using IVF underwent cesarean deliveries (compared with 29 percent of all other births). Compared with 62 percent of women who gestated twins following spontaneous conception that had surgical deliveries, mothers of twins who conceived using IVF faced a 76 percent rate. The comparisons are similar even with singleton pregnancies conceived through IVF: nearly 44 percent of women who conceived using IVF and had singleton pregnancies underwent cesarean section, compared with 28 percent of women who had singleton pregnancies following spontaneous conception (Sullivan et al. 2010).

Because of these risks, the American College of Obstetricians and Gynecologists recommends informing couples of the obstetric and neonatal risks of multiple gestations, so that prospective parents may take this into account when making decisions regarding the number of embryos to be transferred. Yet there are several problems with this suggestion. I interviewed numerous couples who expressed an explicit desire for twins. Indeed, with the costs and stress associated with ARTs and surrogacy, several mentioned that twin pregnancies were a boon; in other words, a terrific deal at "two for the price of one." Moreover, gestational surrogates have little power to influence the decisions regarding number of embryos transferred; such decisions occur in consultations between the doctor and commissioning parents alone. Indeed, while the Indian Council of Medical Research Draft ART (Regulation) Rules (2010) suggest transferring no more than three embryos to reduce the incidence of multiple pregnancies, doctors frequently noted that these recommendations have no legal force. Medical providers and commissioning clients alike told of how doctors routinely transferred more than three embryos in order to increase the chances of pregnancy. Rather than mitigate the risks associated with ARTs, doctors and clients actively produce the population of surrogates as inherently "at risk" by inflicting excessive medicalization on surrogates' bodies, transferring multiple embryos, and increasing their risk of multiple pregnancies. The excesses of medicalization stem from a suspicion of surrogate bodies as especially "at risk" not only through their subjection to ART treatments but also, as I discuss below, through practices that racialize poor Indian women as inherently risky.

Constructing the Risky Population

Because ARTs remain unregulated and no law governs the use or provision of gestational surrogacy services, comprehensive data on the number of surrogate mothers who have undergone cesarean section are unavailable. However, fertility specialists widely acknowledge that cesarean rates for surrogate mothers are well above the national average. Doctors who facilitated surrogacy arrangements or provided prenatal care to surrogate mothers acknowledged to me that the rates of cesarean deliveries for surrogate mothers ranged from 80 to 90 percent, or that "virtually all" surrogate mothers underwent surgical deliveries. These doctors most commonly cited maternal and neonatal risk due to multiple pregnancy as the main indication for a cesarean.

In spite of the evidence that ART raises cesarean section risk, doctors justified the high rates of cesareans by constructing surrogates as a population of women inherently at-risk. Dr. Mehta met with me in between appointments with expectant mothers at her office in a private hospital known for catering to foreigners and wealthy Indians. When I asked her to describe an "average" surrogate pregnancy, she explained that these pregnancies differ starkly from those of women carrying fetuses spontaneously conceived, beginning with the prevalence of preterm labor:

> The average gestation period is between 30 and 37 weeks. Very, very few achieve 38–39 weeks. Multiple pregnancies is an important cause. Also, they are larger than Indian-size babies. These are all Western babies and Western babies are definitely bigger in size than ours. And there are medical complications because these are all multigravida patients. They've all been pregnant two or three times before. So the incidence of preterm delivery, the incidence of pregnancy-induced hypertension, the incidence of hyperthyroidism, anemia, all of that is much, much higher in these women.

Most doctors agreed, citing the surrogate mothers' high-risk pregnancies and greater incidence of multifetal pregnancy as justification for the high rates of cesareans. Dr. Sinha, a fertility specialist who facilitated surrogacy arrangements for foreign couples, emphasized that 80 percent of the surrogate pregnancies she oversaw resulted in cesarean section, due in part to the high rate of multiple gestations. Moreover, she concurred with Dr. Mehta's comments regarding fetal proportions: "It's the size difference! There is a disparity in size; embryos from larger, Western couples' genes get put into the body of smaller, Indian women. So a lot of them will have big babies and they're not going to come out from below. [The discordant size] leads to higher rates of c-sections." Here, the difference in size fills in for a discussion of racial difference, suggesting that small Indian women cannot naturally carry or birth "Western babies" with "Western genes."

The size difference turns up in commissioning parents' accounts as well, with parents reiterating doctors' claims that a physically small Indian woman could not capably carry a healthy pregnancy to term or to deliver vaginally. Matthew and Anthony, fathers to three daughters born through surrogacy in India, felt troubled following the premature birth of their eldest daughter and referred specifically to the small size of their surrogate (two surrogates simultaneously carried the three children, twins and a singleton, who were conceived with sperm samples from each father and eggs from an Indian egg provider). Both agreed that if they were to return to India to commission future surrogate pregnancies, their priority would be to "get a larger surrogate," saying, "We were shocked at how small our surrogate was. She was probably about 100 pounds soaking wet—and we wonder if this had something to do with our daughter's premature birth." They figure physical size as a form of difference that they can manipulate by selecting a larger surrogate, an unrealistic assumption as more than 40 percent of women in India are underweight when they begin pregnancy (Coffey 2015).

Echoing doctors' claims about the relationship between fetal weight and cesarean delivery, Antara, an agent and former surrogate, explained, "Most women I know have 'cesars'; normally only cesar is done because the children are very big in size. They are all more than three kilos; usually 3.5 to 3.75 kilos." But unlike the doctors I spoke with, Antara eschewed genetic or racial explanations for the size difference, stating, "It is not because they are different. It is because they are given more iron and calcium." Demonstrating a sharp understanding of the impact of good nutrition and prenatal care on the fetus, Antara explained that in contrast to "surrogacy babies," their own Indian "normal babies" will normally weigh less than 2.5 kilograms. Yet in gestational surrogacy, "Even the Indian surrogate babies, they are also heavy. They are also more than 3 and 3 to 4 kilos. This is because of the iron and the calcium tablets."

Doctors and clients, on the other hand, refer to race in euphemistic terms as they highlight physical differences between Western clients and Indian surrogates in terms of size and genes, not race. Such explanations rely on essentialist understandings of race and inheritance, further biologizing race and racializing biology (see Thompson 2009). Discussions of size and genes not only reify racial difference, but they also reify the heritability of race through the transmission of genetic material. This genetic material ostensibly carries information related to perceived racial characteristics (such as physical size). By inscribing medical risk through the language of race and genetics, doctors and clients construct the body in terms of the risks it bears. They racialize the surrogate body as an inherent source of risk due to its size. In doing so, they justify the categorization of certain bodies as deserving of certain treatment through perceptions of bodily difference along ethnoracial lines. Doctors construct surrogates' bodies as naturally requiring excessively medicalized care, suggesting that when (similarly raced) Westerners carry "Western babies," medicalized treatment is not necessary.

This construction not only ignores the medical evidence that ART alone—and ART with multiples in particular—imposes a risk of cesarean section. It also discounts the evidence that higher Western birth weights reflect gestation and nutrition, not racial characteristics. Great disparities across the globe in babies' average size at birth have led some researchers to believe that race or ethnicity accounts for disparities in newborn size among different populations. Yet recent studies demonstrate that newborn babies are actually very similarly sized around the world when their mothers receive adequate prenatal care. What matters is not the child's racial/ethnic background or genetic makeup, but the gestational mother's educational, health, and nutritional status (Villar et al. 2014). Similarly, in a study investigating the relative role of environmental and genetic factors in determining birth weight following egg donation, researchers concluded that gestational weight and the weight of the recipient were the primary factors that significantly influenced birth weight. In other words, the birth mother's environment, rather than the egg donor's genes, influenced birth weight (Brooks et al. 1995).

Moreover, racializing the population of surrogate mothers as naturally small (and that of Western clients as naturally large) erases the social and structural factors that influence population height and weight. While research has demonstrated that genetics plays no role in birth weight, a recent study of pregnant women in India found that 42 percent of Indian mothers are underweight, compared with 16.5 percent in sub-Saharan Africa, where children are much poorer, on average, than Indian children (Coffey 2015). The study suggested that a number of social and environmental factors—including gender discrimination, exposure to infectious disease, poor sanitation, and poor diet—rather than genetic or racial differences, shape Indian women's poor health during pregnancy. In the context of justifying high rates of cesarean deliveries, these findings give the lie to the construction of surrogates as being able to "naturally" birth only certain kinds of babies, and to its erasure of the structural and environmental factors that determine fetal size and birth weight.

Ultimately, racialized discourses about body size serve to unify the population of poor pregnant surrogates. Doctors thus can describe

them as a "population" requiring excessive medicalized care. As Khiara
Bridges notes in her discussion of the "Alpha patient population" of poor
pregnant mothers at Alpha Hospital in New York City, "'population' pre-
supposes some significant shared characteristic, and, by implication, a
certain degree of homogeneity" (2011, 155). In this case, the idea that
all poor Indian women are small (and thus incapable of birthing large
"Western babies" vaginally) provides a baseline of similarity from which
a population emerges. Size ultimately functions to blur distinctions
within the group, eliding multiplicity and erasing diversity. Once doctors construct this "at-risk population," they further constitute it through
excessive medicalization, increasing the risks the surrogate endures.

When Dr. Mehta noted the risks associated with multifetal pregnancies and multigravida patients (women who have been pregnant more
than once), she demonstrated this dynamic. As she explained, "Most of
the deliveries are cesarean because they're multiple pregnancies and the
normal presentation is weaker. Most of them are scheduled, especially
with twins." On the day we spoke she had three surrogate deliveries,
all of which were twins born to surrogates who had severe pregnancy
induced hypertension. A number of doctors cited twin pregnancy as a
contributing factor that leads to surgical delivery, as cesarean section
rates are higher for twin pregnancies than singleton pregnancies around
the world. However, studies have found no significant differences in the
risk of adverse neonatal outcomes between women with twin pregnancies who underwent planned cesarean section and those who underwent
planned vaginal delivery. A 2013 study concludes that planned cesarean delivery offers no benefits for twin pregnancies as compared with
planned vaginal delivery (Barrett et al. 2013).

Moreover, doctors admitted that nonmedical reasons contributed to
the high cesarean section rate among surrogates. Sometimes these reasons were couched in terms of risk to the child or surrogate. Doctors
explained that they performed cesareans "at the slightest risk" of something going wrong, implying that they did not weigh the inherent risks
of surgery when deciding on a cesarean. To be sure, surgical intervention
is justified under circumstances such as breech presentation, obstructed
labor, or suspected fetal compromise. Yet the decision to perform a cesarean section is also strongly related to nonmedical factors. Scholars have
argued that nonmedical reasons account for the soaring rates of cesar-

ean, including doctors' preference for the procedure due to convenience, financial incentives, and fear of litigation (Hopkins 2000; Belizán et al. 1999). Higher rates in private hospitals suggest that higher billing rates for operative deliveries influence doctors' recommendations (Potter et al. 2001). A study conducted in India argues that physicians' financial interests determine cesarean outcomes (Mishra and Ramanathan 2002).

Doctors also admitted performing elective cesareans for the "convenience" of the commissioning parents or themselves. Doctors explained matter-of-factly that they induced surrogates' labor to accommodate parents who traveled internationally and were "waiting around" for their child to be born. As Dr. Sharma, a Delhi-based fertility specialist, explained, "A lot of parents will come here and they are waiting for the baby to be born. You can't have them hanging around here indefinitely for three to four weeks. So the labors are induced. In that case, they usually end in cesarean." Dr. Sinha agreed:

> A lot of the cesareans are done simply because of convenience. You've got to give people dates. . . . I usually tell the parents to come down by 37 weeks. They come, they hang around for a week, she goes into labor—well then, good. But if she doesn't go into labor, then we go ahead and plan it. Either plan an induction or a planned c-section depending on the weight of the baby. But it has to be a little different from the routine. You can't just wait—for three weeks the couple is just going to sit around over here, and then wait for paperwork and then go back? It's too much time.

These comments betray no concern for surrogates' medical health or well-being. While at other times doctors claimed they recognized the risks that surrogates bear, subjecting surrogates to high-tech births in the absence of medical justification reveals a lack of regard for their patients.

Commissioning clients also emphasize convenience. Laura, the U.S. mother of three children born through surrogacy in India, said, "Almost all of the surrogate mothers in India have c-sections. It's just easier, less problems. The doctors schedule them. The doctor, she usually c-sections the baby; the head comes out perfect, there's none of this waiting around for them to go through the whole birth process. It's less time. That's the bottom line."

Performing cesareans for reasons of convenience illustrates the ways in which doctors' and parents' desires supplant the health risks surrogate mothers bear. As Dr. Sharma noted, "Cesarean is very high in surrogate pregnancy, because these pregnancies are very aggressively monitored. The slightest chance that there might be a problem, we don't want to take a chance, so we do a cesarean. Because we know the effort that has gone into this." Doctors deem the fetus in surrogate pregnancies especially precious "because we know the effort"—that is, commissioning parents' emotional and financial investment in the fetus the surrogate carries. This approach clearly prioritizes commissioning parents' consumer desires over the health risks to the surrogate mother. It also demonstrates the ways in which racialized bodies intersect with commercial value. Doctors deliver medicalized care under the justification that surrogates' pregnancies are inherently high-risk. Further, they construct the fetuses surrogates carry as more precious than fetuses who share the surrogates' racial/ethnic background, such as the surrogates' own previous pregnancies.

Yet despite the risks involved in cesarean delivery, doctors do not always convey these risks clearly to the surrogates. Dr. Sinha acknowledged that surrogates have "a huge fear of c-sections," which she said they heard about from other surrogates. When I asked Dr. Sinha how she described the risk to surrogates and how she tried to alleviate their fears, she replied, "I tell them I myself have had two c-sections and look at me; I am fine." She acknowledged that surrogates had good reason for their fears:

> The recovery from c-section births is much longer and more painful than vaginal births—you can't walk around, it's hard to move. Women who have never had their own children before have nothing to compare this to. But most surrogates have had their own children through vaginal childbirth, so for them, the c-section is much worse and more painful.

Nonetheless, Dr. Sinha failed to acknowledge the risks of surgical deliveries. By invoking her own reproductive history, she underplayed the risk of multiple cesareans, glossing over the fact that each subsequent operation carries increased risks. Given that many women I interviewed said they planned to act as surrogates again in the future to maximize their earnings, this omission was germane as doctors frequently turned away would-be repeat surrogates because of their previous cesarean sections.

Dr. Sharma, who, like Dr. Singh, worked directly with commissioning parents to connect them with surrogates, acknowledged that cesareans imposed a burden on surrogates:

> I don't charge extra for a twin pregnancy. A pregnancy is a pregnancy. None of my surrogates gets extra compensation. But a surrogate gets extra compensation for a cesarean section. . . . Because for the surrogate, it doesn't really matter whether you're carrying a singleton or twin. What matters is if she's had an easy vaginal birth, then she can return to her normal life within days. If she's had a complicated cesarean birth, it will take her at least a month to recover. That's loss of wages for her, for her husband, problem for her family, so in that case we give an extra compensation even if she has carried only one baby.

In these remarks, Dr. Sharma specifically tied bodies to markets and labor, structuring surrogates' payments according to the type of pregnancy and delivery. She justified the high rates of cesarean by the higher payment: "Cesarean is not that hard to recover from; and with cesarean they are well compensated." Here she diminished surrogates' heightened risk and postoperative pains, emphasizing surrogates' economic incentives as compensating for a cesarean that may not be medically necessary. Dr. Sharma framed the costs of a cesarean in exclusively economic terms, focusing on the surrogate's loss of income and its impact on her family, as well as the higher rate of compensation she received. In doing so, she elucidated the relationship between bodily labor and commercial value that is at the heart of commercial surrogacy arrangements.

Most women I interviewed earned between U.S.$4,400 and U.S.$5,500 for their work as surrogate mothers. Some clinics, unlike Dr. Sharma's, increase the compensation by between U.S.$550 and U.S.$650 for twin pregnancies; the additional compensation for a cesarean typically ranges from U.S.$1,000 to U.S.$3,000. Women gave these figures a good deal of thought in calculating their reproductive labor potential. While some women hoped for twin pregnancies in order to maximize their earnings from a single pregnancy, others, especially younger women, hoped a singleton pregnancy would minimize their risk of a cesarean and maximize their chances of being accepted for a subsequent gestational surrogacy. Indeed, as many doctors and surrogates explained, some women were in extreme financial need, and would readily dismiss the slower recovery, increased pain, and more time away from family, among other outcomes that research links to cesarean sections (Clement 2001; Mutryn 1993). Most doctors, in choosing to diminish the physical risks associated with a cesarean and not to discuss outcomes such as maternal pain or grief, cast these concerns as insignificant. As Claire Wendland states, "The mother's experience of birth and its aftermath vanishes from analysis" (Wendland 2007, 222). Addressing Wendland's call to include maternal subjectivity in analyses of birth and labor, I turn below to the narratives of women who describe their thoughts, concerns, and experiences of pregnancy and cesarean as surrogates.

Policing the Body in Pregnancy

The prenatal care that women receive as surrogate mothers is delivered within a technological, biomedical paradigm of pregnancy, illustrating the contradictory nature of stratified reproduction. Surrogates typically had sporadic access to prenatal care at resource-constrained public hospitals in their previous pregnancies. In their commissioned pregnancies, on the other hand, Indian surrogates receive vast amounts of expensive and technologically driven prenatal care at world-class hospitals. However, while medical providers and most clients praise the high levels of care that surrogates receive, some commissioning parents questioned whether such levels of care were appropriate. Matthew and Anthony, for example, speculated that the stress of all the "routine" tests and scans had negatively influenced their surrogate's health without good cause. As Anthony stated, "We didn't need to see all these scans so often, and I think it must have been stressful for our surrogate to do these tests and scans every two to four weeks." Both Matthew and Anthony implied that such practices had been undertaken for their peace of mind rather than the health of the surrogate or the baby.

Throughout their pregnancies surrogates receive the nutrition, vitamins, and prenatal visits typical of wealthier women's pregnancies. They noted that they never had this level of care when they were pregnant with their own children. This differentiation calls attention to a society that does not value women's reproductive capacities when they bear children who will live in their own families. The Indian state articulates this itself in its messages about population growth and ideal family size that emphasize fertility control (Chatterjee and Riley 2001). Many surrogates had undergone tubal ligation in obeisance to those messages. At the same time, it is their very role as reproducers that grants them access to a new and profitable enterprise in the global economy. Women's narratives reveal that their surrogate pregnancies are overmedicalized in the service of degrading social and medical control, in which women's bodies are closely monitored to ensure their acquiescence.

Surrogates' engagement in prenatal care was vigilantly policed and directly tied to their pregnant bodies' commercial value. Antara described it this way: "The iron and calcium tablets are for weight gain. If the weight does not increase, the doctors ask for the checks back. If the baby is not weighing so much, they cut the surrogate's payment. They can tell you in the sonography how much the baby weighs and they also check the surrogate's weight on the scale. So they say, we have given you protein, we have given you all these tablets for the baby, you need to have greater weight." Swati, a surrogate, agreed: "Yes, they ask us to stand on the scale; if the weight is not enough they cut our salary. One thousand rupees, sometimes two thousand, or three thousand." Antara went on to recount the story of a surrogate patient, Sonal, who was encountering trouble keeping up her weight:

> Madam stopped her checks, as she was not gaining any weight. So at her next weight check she tied stones weighing 2 to 2.5 kilograms to her sari, from here (gesturing at her waist) down. She tied the stones there to show she had gained weight, thinking that she would then start getting her payments again. Then, as the assistant was taking her weight, he tried to push her sari on the side and felt something. The assistant told the nurse that something fishy is going on here. Then they took her inside the doctor's office and found that the stones were tied below down there.

Surrogates' payment is linked directly to their bodies' performance. This reduced pay represents the negative of premiums for bearing twins or undergoing cesarean section. Some doctors have also reported paying surrogates less than the full payment for delivering babies preterm, which reflects the idea that surrogates are being paid for a "product" of determinable quality.

Yet doctors also impose social control on surrogates in terms of their housing and movement, illustrating the intersection of power and mobility in the context of transnational surrogacy (Deomampo 2013). Housing options varied depending on the surrogacy clinic; while some doctors insisted the surrogates move to surrogate housing, others claimed it was not compulsory. Some surrogates encountered conflicting policies with their doctor. Swati claimed that her doctor had not required her to move to surrogate housing. Yet later in our interview she revealed that her doctor had compelled her to stay in housing against her wishes from her fifth month of pregnancy, saying, "I would have stayed at home. Why would I stay in the surrogate housing? I had no choice." She went on to explain, "The housing is not compulsory, but those who have problems must stay there. In my case, I had left to go to my village to attend a family wedding. Because of this Madam [the doctor] said, if you travel to other cities, then your health will suffer. Now you will have to stay at the surrogacy house so you do not keep running away to villages." While doctors claim that women move to housing where their needs are met and they can relax without having to worry about household chores and responsibilities, in practice they use surrogate housing to restrict women's movements, as in Swati's case. Such practices effectively render the surrogate's body an object of surveillance so that she can be available and held accountable at all times.

Ultimately, medicalizing surrogates' pregnancies and forcing them to live in housing the doctors provide serve the same aims: social control and easing the anxiety of commissioning parents. My respondents largely accepted these aspects of their surrogacy experiences, albeit with some ambivalence and frustration. Their feelings about cesarean sections were less accepting.

Surrogates' Experiences of Cesarean Delivery

When I first met Nadia, she was five months' pregnant, her growing belly barely visible beneath a pale pink *salwar kameez* and cream-colored *dupatta*. She was living with her two small children in a tiny apartment provided to her by her surrogacy agency for the duration of her pregnancy. Nadia was born and raised in an industrial city less than forty miles outside Mumbai, and because of her family's lack of financial resources she was unable to complete more than one or two years of primary education. She met her husband in an arranged marriage at fifteen, and had her first son at eighteen. When Nadia gave birth to her second son three years later, she knew her family was "complete." The family was not impoverished as her husband earned a small income as a security guard, but his work was irregular and at times Nadia found it difficult to make ends meet. She learned about surrogacy through a friend, herself a former surrogate, who explained the process and how much money she could earn. Nadia convinced her husband to allow her to try to become a surrogate and following a battery of medical exams, hormone injections, and ultrasound scans, Nadia became pregnant on her first attempt. The only thing she knew about the commissioning parents was that they were not Indian.

As we talked about her experiences with the pregnancy, our conversation shifted to Nadia's understandings of surrogacy. I asked her how the doctor explained the surrogacy process to her, particularly with respect to medical information. Nadia replied, "She told me briefly about the procedure. She said that I have to take injections and a lot of medicines. . . . The doctor really didn't tell us anything. The only thing she told me is that she is going to put three or four eggs of a donor in me. Some women get pregnant and deliver one kid, others will deliver twins." At the time, she explained, her main concern was with becoming pregnant. Once she was confirmed pregnant, Nadia found the hormone injections the nurse administered to support the early pregnancy very painful, although she got used to them. She said, "But now I'm really afraid of my death. The doctors are talking about the possibility of cesarean. This really haunts me more than anything." When I asked if Nadia had spoken with the doctor about her concerns, she replied, "I talked with my friend about it. She has gone through the process and told me not to worry about it. She said that I won't even know when it starts and when it ends." This reliance on social networks to cope with concerns about cesarean section was typical. Eventually, Nadia conceded, "I am so tense; but I think it's time to let things happen in their way. There is nothing we can do."

Nadia's fears of dying are not particularly well-founded; cesarean section is not as safe as vaginal birth but it is nonetheless very safe. If she had had a trusting relationship with her doctor, she might have been able to let go of these fears. But if she had had a trusting relationship with her doctor she might have been able to avoid a cesarean—or to know that she would only have one if it became medically necessary. When she said, "There is nothing we can do," she suggested that surrogates had little recourse to refuse medical treatment. As Amrita Pande has argued, there is a disciplinary project embedded in the surrogacy process that aims to produce "the perfect surrogate—cheap, docile, selfless, and nurturing" (Pande 2010, 970). Nadia's understanding that she had to submit to the range of medical interventions imposed on her in order to support her own family reflects Pande's description of the disciplined "mother-worker subject," who is simultaneously a trained factory worker and a virtuous mother. Her friend's description that Nadia "will not even know when [the surgery] starts and when it ends" reflects an experience common among surrogates in which doctors withhold information from surrogate patients.

Mandira, a twenty-seven-year-old surrogate mother, echoed Nadia's concerns. Together with my translator, I met Mandira for lunch at the cafeteria of Motijheel Hospital, a private hospital in the suburbs of Mumbai in which many surrogate mothers received prenatal care and underwent childbirth. Mandira was talkative and warm, yet appeared slightly dispirited as we ate lunch together. She explained that due to pregnancy-induced hypertension, her doctors warned her to avoid many of her favorite foods, including *achaar* (Indian pickles) and *nimbupani*, a sweet and salty lime drink. Mandira poked at her bland sandwich with some disdain and proceeded to tell me her story.

Mandira met and married her husband when she was sixteen years old; the following year, she gave birth to her first child at seventeen, and had a daughter six years later. Mandira had completed her secondary level education but only managed to find work as a housekeeper. She earned around U.S.$70 per month. Her husband earned the same salary as a security guard, and while the combined salary allowed them to meet their basic needs, they had trouble saving money and Mandira had dreams of sending her children to English-language schools and of purchasing a home. When a neighbor told her about surrogacy, Mandira initially felt that it must involve sexual labor. Understanding the mechanics of IVF reassured her: "This is not a wrong thing to do for any woman." But when I asked how the doctor explained the procedures to her, Mandira replied, "Actually the doctor didn't tell me anything about the process in detail. My friend who took me to the doctor explained the whole thing before going there. The doctor only told me about the financial returns and to avoid sex for a certain period of time during the process." Like Mandira and Nadia, many women asserted that the doctor provided them with very little medical information and that they relied on agents, caretakers, surrogates, and former surrogates in their social networks to convey important information about how to prepare for the medical procedures.

At the time of our meeting, Mandira was seven months pregnant and carrying twins. However, her pregnancy had not been difficult apart from the dietary restrictions. She said, "There's been no actual problem so far for me. I'm just worried about the delivery because if it is not normal, they will do cesarean." She elaborated, "I have two children and both times my delivery was normal. I don't have any idea about how cesarean will be. If they are operating [on] me for the delivery, it will be very painful. And if meanwhile my blood pressure goes up then there's a chance I could die." When I asked whether the doctor had informed Mandira about the risks and procedures of cesarean section, she said, "No, no doctor has offered to do this. But anyway, I already know some things about cesarean, from talking with women in the housing; this is why I'm worried."

Divya, a surrogate five months into her pregnancy, also learned about cesarean and the risks associated with it through her friends, and she too was very afraid. She explained that two women she had met at the clinic had had cesareans and that she feared she might too. "I'm so afraid of that process. I really don't think I'm capable of going through cesarean." She went on to say, "I know it takes lot of blood and it's a major operation as well. You don't understand anything while it takes place but afterwards all the pains of the world are there for the patient."

Padma, a twenty-seven-year-old surrogate who gave birth to twins via cesarean in the year prior to our interview, spoke candidly about the pains she had experienced. Padma turned to surrogacy during a difficult period for her family: her husband had developed problems with his eyesight and was unable to renew the permit he needed to drive the rickshaw he drove for an income. He had taken out a loan to pay for the rickshaw and still had to repay it. As Padma explained, "At that time, we were in great need. My mother-in-law [had just] passed [away], there was nobody to support us, and we had a big loan. That's why I decided to go for surrogacy."

Yet while she had an uncomplicated pregnancy, Padma's doctor scheduled a cesarean section to meet the convenience of the parents who had just arrived in Mumbai. Padma described how she felt following the operation: "I was suffering. My stitches were so painful. And I was not able to get up nor could I sit. It was very painful." In contrast to many women who said that they hoped to do surrogacy again, Padma said she would never do it again. When I asked why, she replied, "If something bad happens to me, then who will look after my children? We have to think about my health, also. I will not be able to do it again." Padma's husband acknowledged, "Surrogacy did help us get out of debt. But it is not to be done again because her health comes first. Money is not that important now."

These stories elucidate the ways in which surrogate mothers cope with their fears and pains related to cesarean delivery; they also reveal how women build communities to share information and concerns. Indeed, Mandira and Nadia lived in the same apartment complex in which six surrogate mothers resided with their families. In this space, their living arrangements served as a key site for building community based on their shared experiences as surrogates. Divya developed her community of women surrogates through clinical encounters. The information the community provided her allowed her to anticipate what lay in store for her during her own pregnancy. The strength the women drew from one another was in contrast to their reported practices of docility in medical encounters. They did not describe themselves as having the right to information or even a say in medical decisions, but they did articulate their economic rights as surrogate mothers.

For instance, at one gathering of around twelve women, surrogates and former surrogates spoke about the kinds of changes they would wish to see in future surrogacy arrangements. They focused on payment and many emphasized that cesarean section should merit more money. As one woman stated, "They should increase our payments—*because if one is going to cut her stomach*, it should be worth it" [emphasis added]. Most women echoed her statement, connecting the "cutting" of their bodies to their right to increased pay. As Aditi explained, "There should be enough money. Our health is also concerned. Because we are giving you a child, we are going to cut our stomach to give you a baby. That means you should also respect our body and also give us enough money. Because after two years you will need us again, but our body will be weak." She emphasized that surgery had long-term health implications.

Others acknowledged that increased pay might not solve all the problems surrogate mothers experienced, and hinted that money could induce surrogates to risk their own health. Jyoti, a former egg donor and now agent-caretaker for surrogate mothers, explained, "Some patients, even if they had cesarean, they will return after six months and say that they need to do surrogacy again. They are in need of money; whatever the way the body may suffer, they will want to do it again." Meena agreed and went on to explain:

> They think we are greedy for money. But some have small children; some may have a husband; some may have a husband but it's as if he is not there. So a woman thinks, "Why can't I try to earn two to two and a half lakhs in seven or eight months?" So, we know that if we take some trouble with our body, it will take care of the education of our children; or we will be able to have a house, so we will be able to live well; or we will be able to satisfy the expectations of our children. This is what every woman thinks. Therefore, if she requires a payment, if she uses her body to earn that payment, then she has full rights over that payment. If she cuts her body, and gives a part of her body, then she should get her rights.

The intertwined experiences of gestational surrogacy and cesarean section clearly articulated to these women the productive value of their bodies, which they viewed as central in their quest to secure their own livelihoods and well-being. Yet while the women's stories coalesced around their intertwined histories of surrogacy and cesarean section, their sense of community was based as much on their social marginality as it was on their biomedical histories. Many of the women I spoke with shared similar economic backgrounds and social histories, as well as common goals: to educate their children, to own homes, and to provide their families with better opportunities for social mobility. In order to achieve these goals they viewed their own bodies in terms of "biovalue," which Catherine Waldby describes as "the yield of vitality produced by the biotechnical reformulation of living processes" (Waldby 2002, 310), and viewed their own reproductive labor as a means of increasing their bodies' biovalue. As the women noted, however, this work comes at a price and the body suffers; the rights they demand, then, are for appropriate and adequate compensation.

In this chapter I've described the ways in which doctors deliver medical care not because it is "best practice" or because they have the best interests of the surrogate in mind, but rather because these medical practices are part of a broader structure that normalizes and naturalizes the hierarchies in which surrogate mothers are positioned as inherently "at risk." The practices of commercial surrogacy and cesarean delivery in India are intertwined in such a way as to effectively erase the surrogate and her concerns from both the pregnancy and the birth. Yet for women undergoing abdominal surgery in order to bear children for wealthier and foreign couples, their bodies become tools for economic gain. On the one hand, doctors often underplay the risks associated with cesarean section even as they highlight those associated with surrogate pregnancy, assuming that women will undergo cesarean section as a matter of course. On the other, while women frequently express fears and concerns about the surgery, they also view their scarred bodies as tools for subverting their marginality and social disadvantage in order to demand economic and political rights. These issues deserve particular attention in countries such as India where the increase in rates of cesarean delivery represents a serious resource drain, particularly as public health remains underfunded. Alongside the unnecessary overuse of surgical deliveries, millions of women who need the procedures do not have access to them, putting their own and their children's lives at risk.

In her analysis of evidence-based obstetrics, Claire Wendland argues that evidence-based calls for cesareans illustrate two core cultural values: safety, which eclipses "selfish" subjective concerns, and market capitalism, "in which long-term complications of consumption are notoriously underestimated when they are imagined at all" (Wendland 2007, 225). Safety and consumer practice, Wendland contends, become embedded in the hospital and embodied in the doctor, such that her expertise represents the safety to be purchased by expectant mothers. As Wendland incisively asks, "How can a conscientious pregnant consumer justify buying anything less?"

In the case of commercial surrogacy, however, the pregnant women are not the consumers with the purchasing power to make decisions regarding a cesarean (or, for that matter, any medical questions dealing with, for instance, the number of embryos transferred or selective reduction). Their bodies become sites of risk and danger from which fetuses (of Western, whiter babies) must be rescued. At the same time, through the biosocial communities that emerge through gestational surrogacy and cesarean delivery, such women view their bodies and their scars as tools for economic gain and social mobility.

7

Constrained Agency and Power in Surrogates'
Everyday Lives

On a sweltering summer day in 2010, I sat in a restaurant on the outskirts of Mumbai with Nishi, a young woman preparing to become a
surrogate mother for a foreign couple outside India. Nishi told me of
how she had separated from her husband four years earlier. Separation
and divorce remain unusual in India, particularly among working-class
women like Nishi, but as one fertility doctor I interviewed explained,
"You'd be surprised at the number of separations and divorces that are
happening [among lower-class women]. . . . After we started doing surrogacy in the past three years, we realized that about 30 to 40 percent
of them are separated." This doctor asserted that most of the women
walked out of their marriages because of abuse and alcoholism; Nishi's
case proved typical.

Following her separation from her husband, Nishi struck up a friendship with Nikhil, a young man from south India who managed an elec-
tronics shop in Mumbai. As their friendship evolved into a romantic
relationship, Nikhil supported Nishi and her two daughters in times of
need. Nishi felt she also should support Nikhil, whom she planned to
eventually marry. When she learned about surrogacy, Nishi viewed it as
a potential financial windfall for her and her family, and began preparing for surrogacy without telling Nikhil. When she told Nikhil of her
surrogacy plans, he disapproved: "He is not agreeing to it. He says don't
do this; he thinks it is illegal. Yet I am trying to convince him somehow
and I am trying. I also told him that everything has been done. I told
him I have done the ET [embryo transfer] and I cannot go back now. So,
he is sitting quietly now, not saying anything." In fact, at the time of our
interview Nishi had not yet undergone embryo transfer. She was still in
the preparatory phases: taking hormone injections and undergoing tests
and procedures to determine her viability as a candidate for surrogacy.
Why was Nishi deceiving Nikhil?

In the context of physician racism and the structural inequalities discussed earlier in this book, how do women challenge racialized constructions of Indian surrogates as docile and virtuous, or manipulative and shrewd? What are the strategies that Indian women contemplating surrogacy employ to negotiate and respond to the structural and social constraints they face daily? How do women enact agency in their efforts to meet or secure their self-defined needs and desires, even as their efforts may maintain structures of inequality? And what are the consequences of such acts of agency, particularly as they challenge cultural norms and expectations? This chapter addresses these questions by tracing the complexities of agency, constraint, and inequality in the lives of women who pursue surrogacy in India. While chapter 5 explored how racial constructions affected women's views of kinship within the families of children born through surrogacy, in this chapter I focus on the ways in which participation in surrogacy affected women's own families and communities.

The views and experiences of women I spoke with resist reduction to simplistic stereotypes and binary oppositions between agent and victim. Indeed, the more I learned about surrogacy in India throughout my fieldwork, the more inadequate these notions became. I contrast the stories of Nishi and Parvati, both surrogates, and their friend Antara, a surrogate agent, whose personal narratives regarding surrogacy and the circumstances that motivated them to become gestational surrogates buttress the point that the global surrogacy industry reflects and reinforces a broader stratification of reproduction. At the same time, however, their narratives reveal the intricacies of women's lives and fend off the temptation to portray them as victims. This chapter shows that surrogate women do find ways to resist racialized constructions of themselves as powerless victims or deceitful manipulators. I argue that in expressing forms of individual and collective agency, the women find ways to challenge gender norms and create new opportunities for themselves and their families, albeit within larger structures of power. As Rhacel Salazar Parreñas has argued in her discussion of migrant Filipina domestic workers' resistance to power (Parreñas 2001, 8), this is the "bind of agency" that Judith Butler articulates (Butler 1997). Because the social processes from which agency emerges limit it, individual or collective resistance do not necessarily challenge structural inequalities. Surrogates tended to highlight their own agency in the process of enabling the formation of new families. Yet while they aim to limit constructions of themselves as victims, they simultaneously note their unequal position in the hierarchies embedded in transnational surrogacy.

However, such expressions of agency also depend on the particular roles and relationships that women play within transnational structures of surrogacy. I contrast the experiences of women who work as surrogates with those who occupy intermediary positions—particularly surrogate agents. Women who act as agents often share the same socioeconomic background as the surrogates and egg providers; indeed, such women are usually former surrogates or egg donors themselves. The distinction between surrogate, egg provider, and agent can be a relatively fluid one, and individual women may move back and forth between these positions or occupy several of them at once. It is not unusual for a woman undergoing surrogacy or egg donation to bring a friend or relative to her doctor; as she receives a commission for this, the woman becomes simultaneously a surrogate or donor and agent. Conversely, agents too might take advantage of opportunities to become surrogates or donors.

In the case of transnational surrogacy, the intermediary position of agent further reinforces structural inequalities, but agents do not always fit the image of the "greedy broker" of whom surrogates are suspicious.[1] In her analysis of the victim/trafficker paradigm used by many governmental and nongovernmental organizations, Warren (2012) has noted how distinctions between sex workers and supervisors are relatively fluid and complicate the image of solo traffickers and victims. From interviews and court cases in Colombia, Warren found that trafficking networks more closely resemble family businesses in which some daughters do sex work while older women find positions as supervisors, and workers and supervisors in trafficking organizations may share housing and meals. Similarly, the agents in my study were often very close to their patients and their families, becoming intimately involved in their everyday lives and family matters.

Notwithstanding these intimate personal relationships, in this chapter I am concerned with the ways in which surrogates and agents occupy distinct subject positions, especially with respect to power and agency. Such intermediary roles illuminate the peculiar contradictions entangled in transnational surrogacy and further complicate analyses of stratified reproduction. As transnational inequalities breed the conditions for a thriving surrogacy industry in India, global processes reproduce stratification itself at local and community levels, creating new categories of actors whose own agency depends on limiting that of others. While women who act as intermediary agents have increased access to power and opportunities that allow them to boost their own social and financial status, their positions simultaneously reinforce the ever more refined hierarchies inherent in transnational surrogacy. By illustrating the diversity of ways in which women enact agency, however limited, through their experiences as surrogates or agents, I highlight the subtleties of intraclass social divisions transnational surrogacy engenders and demonstrate how women both exert power and are subject to it.

Nishi's story was among several that defied my expectations. While there are reports of husbands or in-laws coercing women into surrogacy (De Sam Lazaro 2011), women like Nishi revealed how they asserted their own decisions about surrogacy, often in the face of disagreement and disapproval by their husbands. My focus is on the experiences of surrogates at the local level, depicting relationships among surrogates and their doctors, families, and agents. At the same time, however, it is important to locate these interactions within larger global hierarchies. Clearly, transnational flows of capital, technology, bodies, and reproductive tissues signal how the global surrogacy industry reifies and reinforces global inequities. As anthropologist Rayna Rapp writes, "All of our lives are not only globalized; they are stratified as well" (Rapp 2011, 709). As gestational surrogacy in India necessarily relies on the reproductive labor and bodies of a variety of individuals, it also reveals how stratified reproduction becomes ever more complex with increasing intraclass social divisions among surrogates and surrogate agents.

In what follows, I focus on the experiences and aspirations of women involved in surrogacy, highlighting the nuances of their everyday lives as well as locating their positionalities in relation to local and global hierarchies. Rather than focus on women who lived in compulsory housing (see Deomampo 2013; Pande 2010), I explore women's experiences of surrogacy at home, underscoring intrafamily dynamics and the ways in which women navigate their changing relationships with husbands, children, extended family, and neighbors. Moreover, I critically examine the intermediary positions of surrogate agents, whose roles to date have been relatively understudied, illuminating additional aspects of surrogates' agency and structural constraint. In emphasizing the uneven terrain beneath transnational surrogacy, I want to avoid and go beyond depictions of women who become surrogates as powerless victims in need of aid. Indeed, in contrast to popular media images of helpless women in need of assistance, this chapter illustrates the subtle and explicit ways in which women express agency within the context of structural factors that limit opportunities.[2] Indian surrogates may be or may become victims in the unequal relationships formed between surrogate and doctor or intended parent. Nonetheless, I contend that reliance on the image of the oppressed surrogate neglects the local voices and perspectives long sought by ethnographers and feminists.

A Breeder Class of Women or Unlikely Breadwinners?

Feminist scholars concerned with the impact of ARTs have long anticipated the growth of commercial surrogacy in the global South. Gena Corea, for instance, predicts in *The Mother Machine* (Corea 1985) that white women will hire surrogates of color in reproductive brothels. Janice Raymond, in *Women as Wombs*, describes the growth of reproductive clinics in developing countries that specialize in sex determination, foreshadowing the use of Third World women as surrogate mothers (Raymond 1993). And Barbara Katz Rothman asks, "Can we look forward to baby farms, with white embryos grown in young and Third World women?" (Rothman 1988, 100). As Pande has argued, these Eurocentric portrayals of surrogacy inadvertently reinforce the image of a Third World surrogate as the ultimate victim—of (patriarchal) technology and unequal global power relations (Pande 2014c).

Indeed, beliefs about "Third World difference" play a key role in transnational surrogacy. The surrogate's residence in a developing country strongly influences distorted perceptions of her as "a poor Third World woman of color"; thus, actors perpetuate such stereotypes of a woman oppressed within her own society in a neocolonial context (Banerjee 2010). As Chandra Mohanty has argued, viewing Third World women primarily as victims creates a pattern of domination—a form of discursive colonization—that measures progress against the standard of Western women (Mohanty 1988). In most popular media accounts of surrogacy in India, expressions such as "womb for rent" merge seamlessly with images of the "poorest of the poor" who readily sign up to become surrogates.[3] Yet, such homogeneous images of Third World women who are helpless, oppressed, and thus in need of rescue, predefine women as victims and prematurely rule out any possibility of their being otherwise.

I depart from the premise that all women who engage in commercial surrogacy are exploited victims, a "breeder class" of women who experience severe forms of oppression (see Sloan and Lahl 2014). Instead, as Amrita Pande (2014c) states, "there is a need to recognize, validate, and systematically evaluate the choices women make" in order to participate in the surrogacy industry (9). Like others who have examined women's choices in the context of the sex trade (Brennan 2004; Parreñas 2011; Hoang 2015), I analyze the ways in which women *choose* to become surrogate mothers as a strategy to advance their socioeconomic positions in the local economy. Many scholars of gender have demonstrated how Third World women are frequently misrepresented as victims rather than as women with agency whose desires and motivations guide their decisions (Lynch 2007; Mahmood 2005). I expand on this work to illuminate how surrogates act as astute wage earners—or "embodied entrepreneurs" (Rapp 2011, 710)—within structures of racial and gender inequality.

However, in attending to these experiences of women involved in surrogacy, so too must scholars acknowledge the constraints on women's ability to make "good choices." Bailey (2011) cautions against a narrow focus on choice, which "occidentalizes Indian surrogacy work" (8). Indeed, a single-minded concern with choice "obscures the injustice behind these choices: the reality that, for many women, contract pregnancy is one of the few routes to attaining basic social goods" (Bailey 2011). Women who seek to become surrogates—who negotiate with their families to gain control over their own reproductive potential in order to participate in surrogacy—are unlikely breadwinners who face constrained options in their particular life circumstances. Contextualizing such choices as a form of "constrained but real agency" (Rapp 2011, 11) allows for a systematic evaluation of surrogates' choices in order to uncover the complex structures of power within which they live.

Gender, Reproductive, and Family Relations in India

In order to examine how women enact agency in the context of transnational reproduction, this chapter builds on historical and ethnographic studies of childbirth, reproduction, and reproductive politics in South Asia (Ahluwalia 2008; Arnold 2006; Jeffery, Jeffery, and Lyon 1989; Hodges 2006; Papreen et al. 2000; Ramasubban and Jejeebhoy 2000; Sundari Ravindran and Balasubramanian 2004; Van Hollen 2003a, 2003b, 2013) by examining how gender and reproductive politics both structure and are structured by a wide set of social relations (Sangari and Vaid 1989, 3). In the context of images of colonized India as a mother debased by the British and images of nationalist men who defend and set her free, women in colonial India were symbols and subjects of the nation, as well as mothers who bore sons for the nationalist struggle and later the independent state (Chatterjee 1989a, 1989b; Sinha 2000, 2006). Concurrently, in the late nineteenth and early twentieth century, colonial and nationalist discourses began to focus on the control and management of childbirth (Van Hollen 2003b).

Within this context, scholars have explored how women make choices about childbirth. Van Hollen (2003a) elucidates how the discourse on modernity, in addition to cultural and socioeconomic factors, influences how poor women in south India choose to give birth. Women do not make these decisions in a "power vacuum by totally 'free' individuals" (Van Hollen 2003a, 208). Rather they engage in multiple degrees of agency, seeking out biomedical birthing options because it gives them a sense of being "educated" and "modern." While some feminist scholars have critiqued biomedical interventions as inhumane and invasive, south Indian women sought these same technological interventions for the sense of power (Shakti) and the developed, modern status they could confer. Similarly, this chapter uncovers how low-income women seek participation in third party reproduction in order to attain economic stability.

Such choices occur within shifting social relations in India and a dynamic global economy. In most parts of India, families remain patriarchal, patrilineal, and patrilocal in structure. Within this context, families regard family dignity, status, and unity as paramount; bringing shame or dishonor to one's family is perhaps the greatest transgression one could commit. Moreover, children are socialized into gender inequalities from an early age. Boys are considered economic assets while daughters are trained to become "good" wives and daughters-in-law (Kashyap 2007).

But household composition is in flux; whereas families previously lived in extended, joint family arrangements, there is now a gradual change toward nuclear family patterns in both urban and rural India. The most recent National Family Health Survey (NFHS) in 2005–06 reported that three in five households in India are nuclear, with a slightly higher proportion of nuclear households in urban areas (63 percent) as opposed to rural (59 percent). While joint family living arrangements previously enabled families to share resources in times of surplus as well as scarcity, changes toward urbanization and industrialization have influenced the shift toward nuclear family living arrangements.

Such changes have a significant impact on gender roles and relations throughout South Asia. The proportion of women receiving formal education has increased since the 1990s (although still less than one in three women have completed at least ten years of schooling in any age group) (IIPS 2007, 57). Anthropologist Laura Ahearn has examined the impact of the increase in women's educational attainment on marriage rituals in rural Nepal. In her ethnography of love-letter writing among young Nepalese, Ahearn (2001) found that an increase in female literacy rates enabled new courtship practices and "love marriages." But they simultaneously reinforced gender ideologies by imposing new constraints and expectations for some women. In other words, social changes resulted in new forms of gendered agency while also reinforcing many inequalities between men and women. Increasing participation in commercial surrogacy too elicits new opportunities for women to challenge gender norms while simultaneously reinforcing the social hierarchies that propel women to surrogacy in the first place.

Similarly, social and economic shifts in contemporary India have led to changes in gendered expectations regarding work and income. With the increasing cost of living and the absence of financial security provided by the joint family system, more and more family members other than the husband provide additional income. Changing attitudes toward the previously accepted division of labor—in which women took care of domestic work and men took up financial matters and work outside the home—reflect increasing acceptance of women having jobs to supplement the family income. Indeed, the paid employment of women has been recognized as key to achieving the goal of population stabilization (Ministry of Health and Family Welfare 2000). Yet data from the NFHS indicate that women are about half as likely as men in India to be employed, and when employed they are only 74 percent as likely as men to earn cash. This varies greatly by occupation: 88 percent of women employed in nonagricultural occupations are paid only in cash, in contrast to 31 percent of women doing agricultural work (IIPS 2007, 76). Against this backdrop, surrogacy work emerges as a viable option for women seeking paid employment; not only do women earn monthly cash payments to provide for their families, but they also receive medical benefits. Yet such work does little to challenge the gendered division of labor; it reinforces gendered hierarchies that depend on women's maternal and reproductive duties and limit women's employment opportunities outside the home.

Women's rights in marriage and divorce have also shifted. Higher levels of education are associated with lower child marriage rates, and child marriage has declined with steady increases in girls' school enrollment since the 1990s. Nonetheless, the rate of decline remains slow: the mean age at marriage persists below twenty, and 58 percent of women are married before the legal minimum age of eighteen (IIPS 2007, 163). In my own study, more than half of Indian women interviewed were married before the age of eighteen. These figures are important to consider in the context of surrogacy and its public health implications, as age at first marriage has a profound impact on childbearing and women's health: women who marry early have on average a longer period of exposure to pregnancy and a greater number of lifetime births.

Young brides are also more susceptible to domestic abuse and within marriage in general, domestic violence is widely accepted. More than half of women in India (54 percent) believe it is justifiable for a husband to beat his wife, particularly if a wife has shown disrespect to her in-laws, or if she neglects her house and children. Interestingly, men are slightly less likely to agree, with 51 percent claiming that abusing his wife is justified (IIPS 2007, 475). Within this context, it was not uncommon for women in this study to speak of domestic violence within their marriages, and several women like Nishi had separated from their abusive husbands.

Anthropologists have analyzed the impact of reforms to improve women's rights in marriage and divorce. In her ethnography of lawyer-free family courts and mediations of rape and domestic violence, Srimati Basu (2015) examines the ways in which alternative dispute resolution emerged as a strategy to empower women in marital trouble. Yet Basu finds that legal reforms to improve women's rights in marital disputes have simultaneously reinforced women's economic and social insecurity. Indeed, such inequalities have even undermined the effectiveness of these reforms. Similarly, while some proponents of surrogacy argue that surrogacy offers women an opportunity to earn significant income as reproductive laborers, such forms of "empowerment" in fact do little to challenge gendered hierarchies. Indeed, for many women their marital relationships became ever more unstable. In what follows, I consider the ways in which surrogacy affected marriage and family relations, providing opportunities to improve women's financial futures while undermining their efforts to challenge the gendered balance of power.

Nishi: Surrogacy and Constrained Agency

Nishi was twenty-seven years old when we met in Mumbai in April 2010. She was married at nineteen in what she called, speaking to me in English, a "love-cum-arranged marriage." As the story goes, Nishi's husband was "in love with her from afar" though Nishi did not reciprocate his feelings at first. His mother approached Nishi's family with a proposal for marriage, and while Nishi's mother believed that the family was an appropriate match at the time, she says her mother has come to agree with her that he is "crazy" and has a drinking problem. Following marriage, Nishi quickly had her first child at twenty; she now has two school-age daughters born a year apart. Nishi and her husband are now separated, and she has filed a case for divorce. Since then, she has endeavored to distance herself from her parents and their burdensome financial problems, while working to support herself and her two daughters independently.

Nishi's story reflected the contradictions inherent in transnational surrogacy, which relies on the reproductive potential of bodies that have long been subjected to patriarchy and population control programs. Nishi's first pregnancy ended in miscarriage before she had her first and second daughters in rapid succession. Her fourth pregnancy ended with an abortion. Nishi would have preferred a longer gap between the two daughters, but her husband "wasn't listening" and desired a son. After her abortion, Nishi knew she did not want any more children and underwent tubal ligation, a common sterilization strategy among my respondents; several women mentioned to me the necessity of having the operation, in defiance of husbands who demanded that their wives produce a son.

These decisions complicate debates around reproductive rights and justice: while women like Nishi undergo operations that limit their reproductive potential for their own families, they later become pregnant for other families. Locating Nishi's story within the specificity of India as well as on a global scale reveals the unique contours of stratified reproduction in transnational surrogacy. On the one hand, India marks lower-class women like Nishi as inferior to middle-class women it links with Indian national identity, and the state has historically sought to limit the reproduction of lower-class women (Chatterjee 1989a). Yet the reproductive tourism industry encourages their reproductive potential when it produces children of "worthy" parents, that is, foreign nationals and upper-class Indians.

With respect to class and social status, household income, and family histories of conflict and turmoil, Nishi was similar to many of the women I interviewed (in Nishi's case, she struggled to provide for two daughters as a single mother separated from an alcoholic husband, while also shouldering the financial debts of her parents). However, unlike most of the women I had interviewed, Nishi spoke English. She was confident, articulate, and inquisitive, and she made a strong first impression. Yet Nishi's education was brief and she attended a school in which Marathi was the primary language of instruction.[4] In a conversation with her friend, Antara, Nishi lamented the structural constraints that limited her educational aspirations:

NISHI: Actually I wanted to become a doctor but my father told me he couldn't afford it.

ANTARA: You can become one now.

N: No, it is financially very difficult. I'll have to attend the classes, which is not possible for me. I can study hard but can't attend the classes. I studied very hard in the seventh standard and got first class but I had to give up school after that [due to financial constraints].

Nishi's seventh grade education allowed her to secure a job at a large telecom company where she earned a monthly salary of U.S.$200. This was where she acquired her English language skills.

Nishi exhibited a profound curiosity about the surrogacy process and the risks involved, both physical and legal, particularly in comparison with many women who felt unable to pose questions to their doctors about any aspects of the surrogacy process. Describing how she came to accept surrogacy, Nishi relates:

> My friend, Shanti, told me about the idea of ET [embryo transfer] and I was surprised. By that time, I was aware about the test tube baby but this [surrogacy] was new for me. I thought about it for one month. Then I had a quarrel with my brother. . . . That was the decisive moment for me.

Nishi had been staying with her brother; she was hoping that surrogacy would offer the means to move out.

> I called Shanti and told her that I'm ready for the process. After visiting the hospital, I went to an Internet café and searched for information about surrogacy to prepare myself for the process. Most importantly, I'm earning a substantial amount for my kids. In India we rarely get the chance to earn this much at one go.

In contrast to many women, Nishi took steps to educate herself about surrogacy. She was the only woman I interviewed who mentioned conducting Internet research in order to learn more about the risks involved in surrogacy.

Yet once Nishi began the surrogacy process, her relationship with Shanti soured. Shanti herself had wanted to become a surrogate; she had undergone embryo transfer three times with no success. She decided to become an agent herself and her discussions with Nishi were in her mind related to that. After accompanying Nishi to the doctor where she underwent blood tests and ultrasound scans, Shanti demanded a commission—approximately U.S.$45, which would be deducted from Nishi's payment of U.S.$220 at the time of embryo transfer—for introducing Nishi to her doctor. Nishi's first reaction, as she sat in the recovery room following her initial blood tests and scans, was "Well, if she hadn't told me about this, then how would I have known? I would have had no idea about this." But she later balked at the idea of paying Shanti out of her own earnings. Nishi explained, "She is such a careless agent. I was dying here in the first two months [of pregnancy] with vomiting and she didn't come at all. That's not done."

Nishi's comments illustrate the impact of agents' intermediary positions on surrogate experiences as well as the subtle ways in which social relationships change in the context of surrogacy. As Shanti's focus moved toward becoming an agent, she alienated Nishi. As I will discuss further in the following section, the agent plays a large role in surrogate women's experiences in ways that both enhance and constrain surrogate's opportunities. In Nishi's case, though she tried to learn about the practical details of surrogacy, she still found herself in a vulnerable position as a surrogate, as her agent demanded payment and neglected to care for her in the early months of her pregnancy.

Throughout our meetings, housing was a constant stress for Nishi. When we first met, she was still staying with her brother; according to Nishi, the house was inadequate and she desperately wanted a home of her own. Then her brother's family kicked Nishi and her children out and they had to move in with her aunt, who looked after her children when Nishi was unable to, and lived in a city approximately eighty kilometers outside Mumbai. The uncertainty made it impossible for Nishi to enroll her daughters in school.

Nearly all the surrogates with whom I spoke reported a lack of transparency and power in negotiating contracts. This process perhaps illustrated more than any other aspect of their experience the social and structural inequalities that both propel them into the surrogacy industry and circumscribe their experiences within it. For Nishi, like most surrogates, the experience of signing the contract was confusing and mysterious, and despite her assertive nature she could not advocate on her behalf:

DD: Can you tell me about the contract process?

NISHI: The contract was in two copies, one is original and the other was Xerox.

DD: Did you ask for a copy for yourself?

N: No, actually I wanted one copy for myself but I didn't dare to ask for one. In fact I don't prefer to sign any contract without knowing it in detail but one page was also blank which I signed; also the amount was not filled in. And most importantly she didn't give us a chance to read the agreement. She was turning the pages very fast. If she had let me read the document, I would have read it quickly because I can read English and I can read fast.

While Nishi reported these objections to me, she said she could not speak up in front of the doctor and lawyer who were present when she signed. Indeed, this came up again and again in interviews: surrogates would not confront doctors and lawyers on crucial issues related to their payment for fear of losing their contract. They said that doctors often hinted at an ample supply of women ready and willing to take their place as surrogates, clearly signaling the class issues at the core of the Indian surrogacy industry.

These obstacles notwithstanding, Nishi endeavored to express subtle and explicit forms of agency within these larger structures of power by taking steps to read and conduct research, and independently making her own decisions about surrogacy. Yet despite her own confidence and self-education, Nishi's possibilities for agency remained constrained due to her position in relation to doctors, agents, and other actors involved in transnational surrogacy. In contrast, the story of Antara, whose socioeconomic status was similar to Nishi's but who worked as an agent, uncovers a distinct set of possibilities for agency and power.

Antara: Power and Agency in Agent Work

My research took me into the homes and lives of various surrogates, egg donors, and agents in Mumbai, and as I navigated the anthropologist-informant relationships with each, perhaps the person I am most indebted to is Antara. Though several agents participated in my study, I met with Antara more than any other agent throughout my research. Antara is outspoken and bright, and welcomed me into her home numerous times; a superb host, she unfailingly ensured I was properly fed before "getting to work." She introduced me to the many women she looked after in her role as surrogate agent, and I saw how strong a force she was in their lives.

While her husband, Rahul, had the equivalent of a seventh grade education, Antara had reached the tenth grade, higher than many of the women I had met during my research. In general, the surrogates and egg donors who participated in my study had low levels of education; many stopped school by seventh grade. Yet my study also included a number who had studied up to tenth or sometimes twelfth grade, and some were currently pursuing studies in nursing or cosmetology. Further, while many participants reported financial instability, only a handful of women described themselves as "desperate" for the money; others depicted a solidly middle-class lifestyle. Indeed, despite the financial hardships recounted by most of the women I interviewed, they tended not to be the "poorest of the poor." A few women, like Antara, demonstrated a range of skills that allowed them to capitalize on and negotiate their social positions, reflecting the uniqueness of women who participate in the surrogacy industry and then go on to become successful agents.

Antara and Rahul had two children, a fifteen-year-old daughter and a thirteen-year-old son, with whom I enjoyed chatting in English, playing games, and discussing books and recent movies. Rahul worked for a private company laying roads; for this work he earned a monthly wage of U.S.$110, but since such seasonal work was irregular the family often found itself struggling to get by. When we first met, Antara was thirty-six and described herself as a "housewife"; however, over the months I came to know her and her family, I watched as Antara's work as an agent grew into a job that took her all over the city, into women's homes, doctor's clinics, and hospitals.

Antara's introduction to the surrogacy industry took place several years prior to our first meeting in 2010. When her sister-in-law, Sumita, told her about surrogacy as an income opportunity, Antara initially thought, "What are you talking about? I thought it was probably wrong, but then I realized that I've had my two children. I'm donating something." Rahul, however, did not support the idea, and Antara called on her elder sister and sister-in-law to convince him. Confronted by these determined women of the family, saying, "Look at your living conditions; you need something better," Rahul eventually agreed. Indeed, many women told me similar stories of needing to persuade their husbands to allow them to become surrogates,[5] contradicting concerns among opponents of surrogacy that husbands or other family members coerce Indian women into becoming surrogates.

Antara became pregnant and gave birth to a boy via cesarean section. For this work, she earned around U.S.$2,700, which, in Antara's words, "is not enough."[6] Antara and Rahul put away some of the money for their daughter and used the rest to repair her family's home in the village. In Mumbai, Antara's family continued to live in a rented home.

In 2009, she came to work as an agent for Dr. Desai who had originally facilitated her surrogacy. In her role as an agent, Antara would bring women interested in egg donation or surrogacy to Dr. Desai, for which she would receive a commission of U.S.$90–180. Charged with everything from accompanying surrogates to the hospital for medical procedures, to ensuring that surrogates receive their medications, agents can receive between U.S.$450 and U.S.$900 for their work throughout the duration of a surrogate pregnancy. As I learned from Antara about her perspectives and experiences with the surrogacy industry in Mumbai, I found that the absence of any laws regulating surrogacy resulted in enormous variability in payment and commercial surrogacy practices. Recruiting agents occupy a unique dual position as advocates for their "patients" and as entrepreneurs of sorts, negotiating their own wages with doctors and patients on a daily basis. Antara herself rarely collected payments directly from her patients. Surrogacy contracts with intended parents typically include a clause that covers recruitment fees; thus, Dr. Desai would distribute Antara's fees after receiving her payment from the commissioning parents.

Initially, Antara would roam around her community and speak with women to see who might be interested in egg donation or surrogacy. Eventually, however, as her reputation as an agent spread, I observed a significant boost in Antara's work. By the end of 2010, all of Antara's "patients" would come to her through word of mouth and most of the women she worked with were distant relatives or neighbors in her community. Throughout the months that I met with Antara, I observed how she came to identify more and more as "agent" than housewife, drawing strength and confidence from her role as an economic provider for her family. She typically had between four and seven patients; at her busiest, Antara could be responsible for up to nine or ten patients at varying stages of egg donation and surrogate pregnancy. Antara viewed her work as a full-time job and conscientiously fulfilled her duties; it was not uncommon for her to be out from early morning to late evening, and she meticulously took notes and kept track of all her patients' medications, payments, and doctor's visits. Responsible for dispensing medications and administering hormone injections, Antara claimed, "I'm also a doctor by practice; I don't have a degree so you can consider me 'half-doctor'!" In addition, Antara grew close to her patients on a personal and social level, and on more than one occasion I witnessed her serve as a mediator and advisor for women and their families, offering advice on how to deal with an abusive husband or mediating between dueling sisters. As Nishi told me, "Antara goes all the way in helping patients with their problems. She has earned the right to ask for money as an agent."

During my fieldwork I noted how Antara's financial situation changed over the course of the year, due largely to her work as an agent. When we first met, she and her family were renting a small, cramped one-room flat; several months later they moved to a more spacious, airy home. By the time I returned to India in 2013, Antara was able to purchase an even larger, two-bedroom home for her family, complete with a washing machine and refrigerator (with a lock to secure the medications she stored for surrogates and egg donors), tangible markers of upwardly mobile class status. Antara and Rahul also saved enough money to send both their children to college, so that they could receive the education that neither Antara nor Rahul could achieve. These significant details reveal the impact of Antara's work as an agent; I observed few surrogates achieve similar goals in their postsurrogacy lives.

It was not uncommon for Antara to confront angry or abusive husbands in ways not typically expected of Indian women. Following Antara's experience as a surrogate, her sister Asha too wanted an opportunity to become a surrogate and earn much-needed income for her family. Like other surrogates in the program, Asha was admitted to the hospital for twelve days after the embryo transfer. Asha's husband visited her in the hospital, and Antara thought he had been made uncomfortable by the hospital's policy barring him entry into her room in order to protect the privacy of others. Instead, he had to see his wife in a more public visiting room. He suspected he was actually being barred entry because Asha was committing adultery. While Asha's husband was fully informed about the surrogacy process and the procedures Asha would undergo in order to become pregnant, he nonetheless became angry, insecure, and jealous, harassing Antara and her family following this misunderstanding. Antara said:

> After that we had so much fighting in the house! . . . He said if something goes wrong I will throw both of you out of the house. He just wouldn't listen. He said, "My wife would not even go to the shop by herself and all of you took her so far away." I waited until morning when he sobered up. I said to him, "How did she get so far away? Didn't she ask you? And how dare you use such words about me?" I said if you say this ever again to her and if you so much as touch her or harm her, you watch it.

I asked, "You threatened him?" Antara replied:

> Yes, I told him not to be a bully. I'm good with those who are good to me but bad to those who are bad to me. This is not wrong. There is nothing wrong in this work. If there was, would I have helped my own sister to do it? Then he started apologizing. He said, "Forget it, I will never say anything about it again." Then he said, "Please don't tell her I spoke like that." But I told her [Asha]. If he could speak to us like that, he would have said things to her too. So I told her this is the way your husband spoke to us. Then she must have confronted him. She is also a very strong woman. And now, he's quiet.

Antara navigated threats and assertions of power in her family. The sudden increase in Asha's earning potential as a surrogate prompted Asha's husband to react strongly to the subtle shift in the balance of power in their relationship. I encountered several women who negotiated tense relationships with husbands who were uncomfortable with the significant incomes their wives earned as surrogates. Moreover, Asha's husband's comments hint at persistent misunderstandings regarding surrogacy and its connections to notions of purity and pollution in India. Despite awareness of the medical procedures involved in surrogacy, Asha's husband insisted that Asha must have committed adultery in order to become pregnant.

Yet, while Antara acknowledged the right of Asha's husband to have the final say in her embodied affairs, saying, "How did she get so far away? Didn't she ask you?" she simultaneously resisted her brother-in-law's threats and called on Asha too to confront her husband, signaling subtle and complex expressions of power and agency within the household. While Pande's work on surrogacy in India sheds light on how women view their husbands' role in surrogacy, often deemphasizing their husbands' contribution and joking about their emasculation (Pande 2009a), she conducted her research mainly with women who lived separately from their husbands in "surrogacy hostels" with other surrogate mothers. In contrast, my study provides valuable insights into the impact of surrogacy within the households of surrogate women themselves, revealing the complexities and consequences of female agency as they collide with gendered cultural expectations of female submissiveness and dependency.

In another instance, Antara explained how she banded with other agents to demand equal payments for their patients. As Antara described the monthly payment plan for Dr. Desai, one of the several doctors she worked with, she noted how surrogates were to receive approximately U.S.$65 for monthly expenditures in addition to monthly payments of U.S.$110 to cover their rent and housing (these payments would be deducted from the total salary of U.S.$5,500 that Antara's surrogates earn for their reproductive labor). Yet sometimes Dr. Desai would give U.S.$45 to some patients and U.S.$65 to others. When Antara and her fellow agents realized this, Antara explained, in an account that called to mind the efforts of labor organizers or activists, "All the agents came together and forced her to give equal payments to everybody. So now everyone is getting $65 as allowance for other expenses."

Yet Antara's role as patient advocate sometimes clashed with her entrepreneurial side, revealing the nuanced ways in which agents must negotiate the two positionalities. Antara's work as an agent was often tenuous and insecure, and she recounted how she coordinated with fellow agents to approach Dr. Desai when their own payments were decreasing:

ANTARA: Last month all us agents, around twenty-five, conducted a meeting with her and we confronted her about her decreased payments to us. . . . She is looking to reduce costs as much as she can, and she is deducting from the agent's accounts. Things like injections, traveling from home to the hospitals for different sonographies used to be paid; these are no longer paid nowadays. We demanded the expenses from her.

DD: Did she give you what you asked for, in the end?

A: No, she gave us her notebook to write down the demands. And there is the problem of patients becoming agents. If a patient is bringing someone else as a patient, she makes her an agent, resulting in a rising number of agents. It creates problems for us, and we can't pressure her for more money. We have asked her not to appoint new agents anymore.

DD: Do you know all the agents?

A: Yes, I know most of them. But when a patient becomes an agent it's difficult to keep track of the agents, as it's difficult to differentiate between patient and agent.

While Antara and her fellow agents demanded higher pay and transparent pay scales, they also raised questions about the doctor's tendency to favor certain agents and patients over others. At the same time, however, their objections stemmed from the fact that patients who sought to become agents challenged their position in the hierarchy among doctors, agents, and patients. In seeking to preserve their own power and positions, Antara and her fellow agents aimed to limit the power of their patients to become agents themselves. Ultimately, however, Dr. Desai did not address any of the agents' demands, and with limited opportunities to find alternate forms of income Antara continued to work for her as an agent.

I was surprised, however, when one day Antara presented me with several pages of computer printouts. With little knowledge of English and having few opportunities to do research or access the Internet, Antara had approached a local vendor—the person who helped her secure identification cards for her patients—with a request to research payments for surrogates. When I asked why she collected this information, Antara replied:

ANTARA: I wanted to know the actual payment to a surrogate from the client. If I know the actual payment it will help me to make the process with patients more transparent which eventually helps me to reach more women.

DD: What are you going to do with this information?

A: I'm not sure yet but if we contact the clients directly, it will be more beneficial for everyone.

DD: Is this possible?

A: Why not? There are a lot of people who have asked me to approach the clients.

Displaying a canny sense of entrepreneurship, Antara imagined that she might eventually be able to reach clients directly, avoiding third parties such as Dr. Desai and increasing financial returns for herself and her patients, however unrealistic this might be.

Yet Antara also understood that particular social and structural factors circumscribed the range of possibilities available for women like her to negotiate their own livelihoods. When I asked her whether surrogates should be able to meet the future parents of the child they were carrying, Antara replied:

It should be absolutely acceptable but the main problem is being capable of having a dialogue with them. The language barrier hampers those who really want to communicate with their couple. Couples from abroad usually speak their own language and it is difficult for many illiterate women to respond. These women are really uneducated. In my sister's case, the couple visited her so many times and really wanted to communicate with her but she didn't utter a word. If a smart and educated surrogate had been there, she would have asked them about the details of the actual payment and other things. But here the patients are totally dependent on the doctor. So any added gifts or payment that might have been given by the client but did not reach its destination cannot be tracked.

As Antara's comments attest, lack of education and lower social status in relation to the doctors and commissioning parents largely shapes surrogates' experiences. Indeed, while Antara acknowledged the challenges posed by language barriers between surrogates and intended parents, her remarks illustrate the factors that limit access to resources and motivate women to become surrogates (lack of education, low socioeconomic status). These very factors restrict women's ability to confront intended parents and doctors and to ensure transparency in surrogate arrangements. Indeed, Antara was acutely aware of the inequalities at the heart of transnational surrogacy arrangements as she worked hard to use her own constrained agency to provide opportunities for herself and her family members.

Parvati: Marriage and Gender Relations

I came to meet Parvati several times during my research, as she was a good friend and neighbor of Antara. Thirty-year-old Parvati had been married for sixteen years and was mother to a fourteen-year-old daughter and twelve-year-old son, who were close in age to Antara's children and often would spend time together. Her husband, Kapil, worked as a rickshaw driver and frequently drove my translator and me to the train station after long days in Antara's home. Kapil sometimes earned between U.S.$130 and U.S.$150 monthly as a rickshaw driver, yet this was unstable employment and the family suffered frequent stretches of financial instability. Parvati had completed some primary school education (fourth grade) and worked as a housewife.

Parvati learned about surrogacy through other women in her community and approached Dr. Desai in the hope that she could become a surrogate. Dr. Desai, however, responded that Parvati's children were too old. "What will your daughter think about you being pregnant now?" Dr. Desai asked. At this point, Kapil was unaware of Parvati's intention; Parvati never mentioned the visit to Kapil.

However, Parvati persisted and eventually convinced Dr. Desai to accept her as a surrogate. When Parvati explained her surrogacy plans to Kapil, he was immediately on board when he learned of the money that she would earn. Parvati, who would eventually become pregnant with twins, would earn more than U.S.$7,000, approximating the amount that Kapil could earn in four years driving a rickshaw. Parvati planned to keep some of her earnings for her daughter's wedding and use the rest to buy a house for her family.

At one of our meetings, in her second month of pregnancy, Parvati seemed fine and easy-going as always. When I asked how the pregnancy was progressing, she replied that all was well and she had no complaints except for the fact that she disliked taking so many medications. She went on to describe the day she underwent embryo transfer:

No problems with the process so far, though we enjoyed a flight to Delhi. We had never been on a plane nor to Delhi before. We had some sweets on the plane, but we didn't have an opportunity to see the city because we were there for one day only. We went directly to the hospital where we had to wait until 5:00 p.m. Then we went through the process [embryo transfer], which was completed by 7:00 p.m., and we took the return flight back to Mumbai the same night.

When I asked with whom she traveled, Parvati explained that Dr. Desai and another woman undergoing embryo transfer joined her on her trip. She was clearly excited about having been on a plane to Delhi, something neither her husband nor anyone in her family had done before.

Parvati went on to describe how her current pregnancy contrasted with her previous pregnancies with her own children: "This is better than the previous experiences. In my own pregnancies, it was for myself, which was obviously an important moment in my life. But this is something different. And also we are doing this because of our poor conditions. We are going to get good financial returns out of this." When asked how her daily routine might be different and what her husband's thoughts were on her pregnancy, Parvati replied, "Yes, it is definitely different. We are more careful this time whereas we used to do all the work with our own pregnancies. We follow all the doctor's instructions, like avoiding lifting heavy objects, etc. My husband feels good because we'll be getting a lot of money. There's been no difference in his behavior for me. He has accepted the process positively."

Yet as her pregnancy progressed, Parvati's attitude would change dramatically. At a subsequent gathering in Antara's home, Parvati, then five months pregnant, was visibly stressed, unhappy, and annoyed. The tension was apparent on her face and she seemed to have trouble relaxing as she sought the advice of Nishi and Antara, who were present that day along with others. In the middle of a conversation with another woman who was extolling the virtues of her supportive husband, Parvati suddenly interjected, in a bitter tone, "If your husband is nice and supportive, then you don't need anything else in the world." My translator, Prachi, gently replied, "Why do you say that? I'm sensing some problems with you, Parvati." Parvati went on to explain, "My husband is very selfish. Generally husbands are not that bad. Sure, everybody is selfish but he has crossed all limits." At this point, Antara remarked:

> He [Kapil] thinks we are planning to send her [Parvati] along with those foreigners. Her husband always thinks I've provided her with some foreign connections. Parvati's health is not good these days. He should understand this and help her with the housework. What she is doing is to benefit his family only. But he doesn't take all these things into consideration and hurts her whenever possible. He always pushes her to handle all the family responsibilities alone. This could create some problems for her in the process. He wants financial benefits but doesn't want to do a single small thing to help achieve that.

Though Parvati claimed earlier in her pregnancy that Kapil remained positive and supportive, clearly her marriage, as well as her health, began to suffer as a result of her pregnancy. Antara observed that Kapil harbored the paranoiac belief that Parvati would eventually leave India (a highly unlikely outcome of Parvati's surrogacy process). He also refused to relieve Parvati of the burden of housework and other responsibilities. Antara was quick to point out that not all Indian men behave that way: "I've given him [Kapil] the example of my husband, too. Rahul also helped me in difficult situations during my surrogate pregnancy. He did all the things like cleaning the floor, washing the clothes, etc."

Later in the day, we returned to discuss Parvati's unfortunate situation in more detail, with both Antara and Parvati elucidating Kapil's various offenses. As Parvati's agent, Antara had much to say on the matter of Kapil's treatment of Parvati. Antara began, "That guy [Kapil] is so bad and corrupt! Whenever Parvati is picking up her payment, he forces his son to leave school and follow her everywhere like a spy to know actually how much she is getting!" Parvati replied, "He thinks that now that I'm getting so much money, I might run away with it. If he continues to behave like this, one day I'll definitely run away with someone!"

Here, Antara picked up and continued to tell Parvati's story, after sending the children who were present out of the room:

> When the actual embryo transfer takes place, the surrogate is keeping someone else's embryo. But he [Kapil] is still under the impression that

to do this his wife has to sleep with another person. He keeps taunting her about this. Doctor has told him all about the process and I've also told him everything in detail. I've explained it with as much detail as possible, more than I've had to do with anybody else, but he keeps harassing her.

When asked what she was planning to do, Parvati simply said, "I'm in the fifth month now. There are still four months to go. I'll have to suffer for another four months like I've done so far. I have to take care that the baby is not affected. It's such a waste of time to speak with him. If he doesn't get it after so long and after so much talk, there is no point in talking with him any more." In the background, another woman, Aditi, quietly commented, "She doesn't even eat on time." And Nishi replied, "We are usually at risk of having this kind of problem in our society because people don't understand surrogacy that well." While her pregnancy was clearly taking a toll on her family and her health (she was missing meals, as Aditi revealed), Parvati remained focused on taking care of the fetus she was carrying.

Parvati's situation illuminates the impact that surrogacy can have on a woman's marriage and family. While some women's husbands understood the process and supported their wives' decision to become a surrogate, Parvati experienced a dramatic shift in her relationship with her husband. As she explained, "We both wished this [surrogacy] for us. He didn't force me to do this. But I think now the money is making him a little overconscious. Even now he's not afraid to raise the question of how can I be carrying the children of only one person, since there are two. I told him in anger that I've slept with two men and am having two embryos. What a stupid person he is." Interestingly, Kapil's reaction, like that of Asha's husband, demonstrates not only a discomfort with Parvati's surge in income but a lack of understanding of the process of surrogacy. These misconceptions about assisted reproduction—namely, that Parvati must have slept with another man in order to become pregnant— also reveal Kapil's assumptions about the violation of women's bodies in the process of surrogacy and call to mind traditional Indian beliefs about purity and pollution in the Hindu caste system.[7] They also reflect the ways in which surrogacy is stigmatized and likened to sex work in the public imagination (Pande 2009b).

Yet when I asked what she planned to do about her husband's behavior, Parvati replied,

> Women here have to stay with their husbands because they can't survive without them. Now that I'm getting so much money he is thinking that I may run away with someone. But I don't think like that. I'm not going to run away and do such things. I have to stay and I want to see my daughter's wedding and all. He even hits our daughter for not listening to him; he thinks I'm telling her to not follow him. And he is training our son to spy on me all the time. But I told him [Kapil] that he's not going to obey you forever. Once he's grown, he will not be yours or mine. He'll be his own person and will use his own mind.

With Parvati's remarkable increase in income, the shift in the gendered balance of power in their relationship provoked Kapil's increasing suspicion and anger not only toward Parvati but toward their children as well. In the end, Parvati remained, as she predicted, with Kapil and her family. Though Parvati earned a significant sum for her work as a surrogate, it was not enough; in order to have the amount needed for the purchase of a home, Parvati had to sell her family jewelry.

Indian women involved in surrogacy take up a diverse set of roles and responsibilities, and in contrasting the relative positions of the surrogate and the agent I have shown how these intermediary roles have resulted in intraclass divisions that engender further stratification among women. In Antara's case, her experience as a surrogate facilitated her ascension to her role as a sought-after surrogate agent, and this role afforded her power and agency, however constrained.

Others have briefly examined the relationships between surrogates and agents, or "brokers" as Pande calls them. In her work, Pande has analyzed how surrogate hostels can represent a powerful site of resistance against brokers. As Pande describes it, the surrogate women banded together and complained to their doctor about the fact that they had to pay their broker U.S.$200 from their own earnings. Eventually, the doctor added a clause to her contracts stipulating that commissioning parents would be responsible for broker payments (Pande 2010). Yet Pande's study, located in a small city in the western state of Gujarat, focused on women whose agents played a smaller role because they lived in a surrogate hostel for most of their pregnancies. Agents played a more significant role in the lives of the women I interviewed, and thus had more power and involvement in surrogacy arrangements. Unlike the agents in Pande's research, they chaperoned women to clinics, administered injections and medications, mediated family quarrels, and disbursed payments. However, while Antara cared about the lives of her "patients," she also sought her own financial future and well-being. I found that incentives encouraged women in intermediary roles to improve surrogates' living conditions and foster their loyalty; at the same time, the incentives prompted agents to protect their own relative positions of power by constraining the agency of others.

In her ethnography of the delivery of prenatal and birth health care in a New York City public hospital, Khiara Bridges (2011) has argued that "the very act of being pregnant" is an act of resistance by poor women who have historically been viewed as "undisciplined breeders" but "'good enough' nurturers to work as childcare providers for other, more privileged class and ethnic groups" (Ginsburg and Rapp 1995, 3). In transnational surrogacy too, the act of being pregnant is an act of resistance to the larger structural forces that constrained their own opportunities as working-class Indian women. Indeed, for women in a society in which they are not primary wage earners, surrogacy represents an enormous opportunity to achieve greater power in financial terms. Yet in challenging such gender norms, women encountered varying responses within their families and communities.

Some narratives, for instance, reveal how their efforts at resistance actually re-created structural inequalities. Though Nishi sought to improve her family's financial future through surrogacy and took proactive steps to educate and protect herself against the risks involved, she remained unable to negotiate key aspects of her surrogacy contract. While Parvati earned many times the income of Kapil, she affirmed that women simply "can't survive without their husbands." Antara too worked to increase payments for her surrogates, yet her negotiations of power as an agent did not represent interventions against structural processes. Rather, her actions intensified and re-created hierarchies among working-class women involved in surrogacy.

In this chapter I have offered a critical examination of the views and experiences of the women without whom gestational surrogacy would be impossible, in order to reveal how women express agency in the context of structural constraints and social inequalities. While focusing on the everyday experiences of women involved in surrogacy, I have connected their experiences with the larger global structures that foster reproductive tourism. The narratives of Antara, Nishi, and Parvati illustrate the unique contours of stratified reproduction in the context of transnational surrogacy while simultaneously challenging popular racialized portrayals of Indian surrogates as powerless victims. While the system treats surrogates as though they are no more than wombs-for-rent, their voices and hopes reveal complex histories of women and families striving to enter the global market on the best terms possible.

Conclusion

When I conducted my fieldwork in 2010, it was a particularly interesting time in the growth of transnational surrogacy in India. By then the practice had gained widespread media attention in India and around the globe, and clinics were working to adjust their practices as they received more international clients. The increasing visibility of the surrogacy industry brought renewed scrutiny as the broader public read about "stateless babies" (Mahapatra 2008) in the media and tragic reports of women like Sushma Pandey, who died after donating eggs (Cook 2012; Janwalkar 2012), and Premila Vaghela, who died after delivering a premature son for a U.S. couple (*Times of India* 2012a). This attention eventually led to the 2008, 2010, and 2012 Draft ART (Regulation) Bill and Rules in India's parliament.

I returned to Mumbai in the winter of 2013 to find that much had changed in India's surrogacy landscape. Earlier that year the Indian government's Ministry of Home Affairs (MHA) took its first step toward regulating surrogacy by requiring special medical visas of all intended parents who travel to India. However, these surrogacy visas stipulated that gay couples, single men and women, nonmarried couples, and people from countries where surrogacy was prohibited were ineligible. Visas would only be granted to heterosexual married couples who had been married for at least two years and who hailed from countries where surrogacy was legal. As the Draft Bill languished in parliament, the MHA's visa requirement prompted much debate about the priorities and desired impact of regulation. While women continued to face physical risks in the treatments associated with surrogacy, many wondered why the government was policing the sexuality of parents who traveled to India (Roy 2013).

Indeed, the composition of commissioning clients traveling to India changed swiftly. While India had previously emerged as a key destination for gay couples and single intended parents, the medical visa requirement, as one doctor stated, had caused "a big blow to everyone's international work." Third-party surrogacy brokers whose client rosters consisted of primarily gay couples and individuals scrambled to find new surrogacy destinations in other Asian countries (Bhowmick 2013). Doctors circumvented the visa requirement by opening clinics or hospitals in neighboring Nepal, where Indian and Nepali surrogates would give birth, while commissioning parents ventured to countries with lax regulations such as Thailand. As the global movements of people seeking surrogacy shifted from one country to another, governments found themselves playing "catch up" as they responded to demands to regulate a rapidly growing industry. Several high-profile scandals focused attention on the unregulated surrogacy industry in Thailand (Fuller 2014), for instance, prompting the government to act swiftly and enact laws prohibiting commercial surrogacy for foreigners (Phillip 2015).

While global shifts in the surrogacy industry rerouted many commissioning clients to other countries, the domestic market for surrogacy services in India underwent significant changes too. As one doctor updated me on her practice, she explained that while she saw a decrease in international clients, her business had not suffered: "My clients are half and half now: half international and half Indian." She went on to describe how high-profile Indian actors and celebrities had helped prompt the increasing awareness and acceptance of surrogacy in India:

> After Shah Rukh Khan and Aamir Khan did surrogacy, I think people became more open to the idea. I had a friend, actually, who I used to run with. He and his wife were seeing an IVF specialist for a long time and couldn't get pregnant. Eventually they decided to come to me [to try surrogacy]. They came here, we did the procedure, and suddenly they get pregnant. So the wife came to me and said, "I was thinking of doing this whole thing, where you can get one of those devices that makes you look pregnant, to falsify your own pregnancy. . . . But you know what, if Shah Rukh Khan can do it, I can do it. So what's wrong with [doing surrogacy]?"

After their surrogate gave birth to twins, the couple announced to their friends and family that they had hired a surrogate, an announcement clearly influenced by the increased attention brought to surrogacy by such well-known actors.

But the visa restrictions coupled with the increase in awareness affected the options available to would-be surrogates as well. While Antara reported encountering an increase in domestic couples in her work as an agent, she also noted that this shift negatively affected surrogates, whose options for profitable surrogacy arrangements with foreign clients had dwindled. Many women saw no choice but to accept lower pay in order to work with doctors who offered "budget surrogacy" packages to Indian couples. While many concerned parties argued that the previous guidelines were inadequate, some feminists claim the Indian government's recent efforts to regulate the industry, including the proposed 2015 ban on surrogacy for foreigners, will only create further opportunities for exploitation (Aravamudan 2015).

As the surrogacy industry continues to change, all these shifts have occurred within a "racialized social structure" (Winant 2004) through which actors develop and rely on racial reproductive imaginaries to make sense of their participation in transnational surrogacy arrangements. Indeed, racial reproductive imaginaries continue to shape how various actors are positioned in the transnational spaces in which surrogacy arrangements unfold; they also govern the ways in which actors give meaning to their relationships with one another. For instance, in April 2015, in the wake of the devastating earthquake in Nepal that left more than 8,000 dead, a story about Israeli parents airlifted out of the country with their newborn babies born through surrogacy prompted much outrage, as many noted the lack of concern for the Nepali and Indian surrogates left behind. As writer Alon-Lee Green asked, "How can it be that none of the human interest stories or compassion-filled posts mentioned these women, who came from a difficult socioeconomic background . . . to rent their wombs . . . who now, like the babies they've just had, are also stuck in the disaster zone?" (Kamin 2015). The story highlighted the ways in which differently racialized bodies are privileged (or not) in their ability to move freely across national borders. It also demonstrated the racial reproductive imaginaries through which certain bodies are deemed privileged or powerless as transnational surrogacy occurs across racial, ethnic, and class borders.

Technologies of Race

Kalindi Vora has argued that we must pay close attention to the ways in which specific technologies "may operate in the service of racializing and devaluing particular populations" (Vora 2015, 142). In this book I have approached transnational surrogacy as a matter of reproductive technology in order to think about what is produced and reproduced, specifically with regard to race. In other words, to view surrogacy as a technology of race is to highlight the process of racialization that occurs through a specific set of practices. It is to understand surrogacy as more than simply reflecting forms of racial categorization, but as a complex site of racialization—a place from which actors "make" race in particular ways.

In this book, we have explored transnational surrogacy as a technology of race by demonstrating how populations can be divided and made distinct in fundamental ways. We have seen the ways in which socioeconomic, race, and class inequalities have come to be considered normal and justified through the naturalization of racialized bodies and the perception that certain kinds of bodies are well positioned to be either consumers or providers of reproductive parts and labor. For instance, while racial hierarchies imbue different shades of skin color with different meanings, the international industry in egg donation normalizes racial and color hierarchies. Certain racialized bodies become characterized as eligible egg providers while others are good womb renters. When the global reproductive market in eggs and wombs makes racial preference appear natural, this pattern of distribution normalizes race (and other genetic preferences) as a commodity to be purchased. Moreover, while commissioning clients often constructed Indian women as naturally qualified to become surrogate mothers or naturally desired as providers of eggs because of their "exotic beauty," the medical gaze of fertility specialists framed Indian women as inherently predisposed to become surrogates because of their behavior, their culture, or their racialized biology. I have argued that such racializations serve to divide and distinguish groups of people in ways that both challenge and reinforce stratified reproduction as reproductive actors make sense of their complicated relationships with one another.

In her discussion of the ways in which race functions as a technology that conceals human beings' relationship to power, philosopher Falguni A. Sheth (2009) bridges what appear to be two fundamentally distinct discourses: that of "biological race," which grounds its arguments in biology, genetics, phenotype, and genealogy, and "political Othering," which refers to the ways in which certain populations have been constructed as foreign or Other. While scholars often view practices of Othering as "not really" about race "because of the nonbiological grounds by which 'Othering' occurs" (Sheth 2009, 24), Sheth suggests that both biological race and political Othering discourses are about understanding populations as different or Other through race. Locating the similarities between these discourses enables us to view certain populations as "the focus of a racialization that does not conventionally resort to eighteenth- and nineteenth-century European classifications of race" (Sheth 2009, 25).

These dual discourses are central to the racial reproductive imaginaries I have described as inherent to the practice of transnational surrogacy. In this book, I have noted the ways in which actors' racial reproductive imaginaries assign meaning to phenotype and biology, imbuing skin color and gametes with notions of exotic beauty and kinship. I have also explored how Western commissioning clients and Indian doctors depend on processes of Othering to construct Indian women as objects of rescue, shrewd entrepreneurs, or risky bodies to be medicalized and controlled. Yet at the same time, I have shown how women attempt to challenge racialized constructions of Indian surrogates as docile, revealing the various ways in which women exert power, however constrained.

Reanimating Stratified Reproduction

By looking closely at the ways in which actors construct notions of race in the context of transnational surrogacy, this book has shown how transnational reproduction depends on racial reproductive imaginaries that naturalize and justify the unequal relationships that make possible transnational surrogacy in India. This approach illuminates several consequences for theorizations of power, inequality, and stratified reproduction. First, by viewing surrogacy through the lens of race, we may begin to challenge the dominant narratives used to explain transnational surrogacy. These narratives focus on surrogacy as an opportunity to make parenthood possible for same-sex and infertile couples, to challenge inequality by empowering women to earn significant sums of money to improve their standard of living, or as a practice that exploits and victimizes poor Indian women. By approaching surrogacy as a technology of race, we may come to understand that undergirding such narratives are essentialized notions of race that maintain structures of inequality.

Moreover, the flexibility of the period of high growth with minimal oversight in the surrogacy industry revealed an opportunity to examine the unstable connections among the various actors involved in transnational surrogacy. A strategic analysis of the racial reproductive imaginaries that people rely on provides insight into the ways that different reproductive actors make sense of their relationships with one another, illuminating the intersections between shifting constructions of race and kinship. Examining how notions of family overlap with race, gender, class, and nation reveals how these systems mutually inform one another. It also calls attention to the ways in which racial imaginaries construct the family in global surrogacy arrangements by highlighting the constellation of sites and actors who make that family. Put another way, attention to the intersections of race, class, gender, and kinship reveals from the very start the nuanced sets of negotiations that different actors embody as they make sense of their participation in global surrogacy. A systematic analysis of these negotiations sheds light on the ways in which these complex networks of actors imagine family, as well as the configurations of power that shape reproductive possibilities and constraints, especially in the context of global inequalities. Understanding the implications of these intersections offers opportunities for refocusing bioethical, health, and policy debates around surrogacy back on the historical and social conflicts that enabled the spread of global surrogacy in the first place. In other words, attention to the overlaps between race and kinship reveal how possibilities for justice might begin just where inequalities are perpetuated. In this ethnography, I have closely examined these intersections in order to propose a more robust and nuanced conceptualization of stratified reproduction that accounts for spaces of resistance and strategies for challenging hierarchies of power within global reproductive networks.

By examining the practice of transnational surrogacy from the perspectives of the range of actors involved, I have elucidated the contradictions and complexities that encompass transnational reproduction. Through this multiperspectival approach, this book has used transnational surrogacy as a lens to understand changing notions of family and kinship, race and relatedness, and power and agency. This work builds on feminist theoretical analyses of reproductive labor and social stratification, particularly within the landscape of global capitalism in the twenty-first century. While many practices and discourses examined in this book are not new, one of the key contributions of this volume is its emphasis on the particular sociocultural, political, and historical contexts that make possible the kinds of transactional relationships I have described in the preceding chapters. Currently, the global surrogacy industry is in a moment of tremendous flux. My focus, then, has been on the relationships of race, kinship, and inequality that have emerged amid complex histories in a specific time and place. From this perspective, this book presents ethnographic findings that shed light on the messiness of "reproductive entanglements" (Rapp 2011) in a particular historical moment, contributing to a growing literature on surrogacy in India and around the world. With the ever-increasing global market for reproductive and affective services, this book holds important implications for scholars who examine inequalities that emerge from transnational linkages, technological advances, and service work. While I have focused on the specific case of transnational surrogacy, the findings of this research can shed light on power and social relationships formed through other "intimate industries" (Parreñas, Thai, and Silvey 2016) such as medical tourism, international adoption, international marriage brokerages, call centers, and sex, domestic, and care work.

By emphasizing the role of racial reproductive imaginaries in perpetuating inequalities at the core of transnational surrogacy arrangements, this book calls attention to the naturalization of race and inequality in order to recognize and challenge the operation of power. These imaginaries also have important implications for public health. The relationship between race and health disparities is well documented, and scholars have shown how racism and other forms of discrimination have profound implications for reproductive health and infant mortality

(Mullings and Wali 2001; Mullings 2005; David and Collins Jr. 2007). As discussed earlier, there are significant risks associated with overreliance on medical interventions, particularly when not medically indicated. This book is concerned with the processes of racialization that influence such interventions, particularly the extraordinarily high rates of cesarean sections, induced labors, and other medical interventions, as well as the high prevalence of multiple pregnancies and preterm births. As shown by the experiences of surrogate mothers, racialized constructions of Indian women also profoundly influence their experiences of surrogacy in ways that make them feel devalued and disrespected. We do not yet know the full impact of such forms of racism and racialization on women's psychological and reproductive health; this book calls for more research on the implications of racism on the health of women and children who experience surrogacy.

More broadly, I have attempted to portray and analyze the lives and experiences of the actors involved in surrogacy, demonstrating the importance of ethnography in illuminating the nuanced ways in which people engage with the structures of race, class, and socioeconomic inequality at the heart of transnational surrogacy. Understanding reproductive actors' lived experiences holds important implications for studies in bioethics and policy making in the fields of human biotechnology. As surrogacy remains a controversial practice, I contend that society must not only focus on the process or act of surrogacy, but also on the causes and motivations of people who pursue surrogacy as a path to parenthood or alternatively, as an avenue to financial security. Thus, I argue for a more political-economic orientation of bioethics, or a "practice-oriented approach,"[1] that takes into account the social, political, and economic contexts of the actors involved in surrogacy.

This grounded approach contextualizes the motivations behind women's desire to become surrogates in the first place. As described in this ethnography, surrogates are not the "poorest of the poor" as commonly described in the media, yet they are indeed struggling mothers and wives seeking an income to alleviate the financial burdens that come with raising a family, sending children to school, and securing permanent housing in Mumbai, where housing is scarce and expensive. We cannot understand why they seek to become surrogates unless we consider the structural contexts that have shaped their lives. Many opponents of surrogacy take issue with the practice because of its implications for the commercialization of reproduction and exploitation of women, among other bioethical implications. These are important issues to consider; however, I would add that the debate should also focus on easing the structural and gender inequalities that limit women's choices and make surrogacy their most appealing work option.

Here, the concept of reproductive justice offers a vital framework for evaluating the structural conditions and circumstances of constraint that characterize transnational reproduction. While the reproductive rights movement historically has focused on notions of choice and privacy, working to protect individual women's rights to reproductive health care services (especially abortion and family planning services), a reproductive justice (RJ) approach aims to change structural power inequalities. The RJ movement, in other words, recognizes that "a woman's lack of power and self-determination is mediated through the multiple oppressions of race, class, gender, sexuality, ability, age and immigration status" (ACRJ 2005, 2). Reproductive justice, then, seeks to ensure that women and girls attain the power and resources to make their own decisions about their bodies, sexuality, and reproduction. As others have argued, viewing surrogacy through the lens of reproductive justice enables us to emphasize the social and economic conditions that constrain women's choices (Bailey 2011; Fixmer-Oraiz 2013). It also prompts important questions about the impact of transnational surrogacy on women's lives; as Sharmila Rudrappa incisively asks, "Transnational surrogacy may afford working-class women the ability to earn some money, but how do these markets in life facilitate their attempts to build long-lasting social and political capital, and lead dignified lives?" (2015, 172). As I have shown, transnational surrogacy indeed offers some women relief from their financial burdens; yet the complex racializations I have described in this book illustrate how transnational surrogacy arrangements serve to reinforce the social hierarchies that enabled the growth of the industry in the first place.

This book shows the importance of how people imagine their reproductive endeavors through ever-changing constructions of race, as well as the public health and bioethical implications of such imaginaries. Moreover, adding a racial analysis to surrogacy arrangements provides social scientists, activists, and other concerned parties with a framework to recognize the diverse and pernicious ways in which power operates in commercial surrogacy. Clearly, reproductive justice cannot be achieved without a keen understanding of the systems of power and oppression present in women's lives. Only with such an awareness might we move toward addressing the inequalities that bolster the surrogacy industry around the world.

APPENDIX

Profile of Study Participants

I collected ethnographic data primarily through participant observation and in-depth interviews with a wide range of actors. In this appendix I describe the different groups of actors who participated in this study, providing broad demographic background information on the research participants.

Commissioning Parents: During the course of this research, I conducted interviews with a total of 46 intended parents (representative of 29 couples and 2 single intended parents)[1] who traveled to India for either IVF or surrogacy. Intended parents who traveled to India solely for IVF were all heterosexual married couples and hailed from Tanzania, Ethiopia, Nigeria, and Myanmar. Intended parents who traveled for gestational surrogacy (with or without egg donation) came from primarily high-income countries: 19 intended parents from the United States and 9 from Australia, with the remaining parents traveling from Norway, France, Canada, Israel, and the Netherlands (in rare cases, individuals held citizenship in countries other than those in which they lived, for example, one British national lived in the Netherlands and sought British citizenship for his children). Of the 39 intended parents (comprising 24 couples and 2 single individuals) who pursued Indian surrogacy, 19 identified as gay. Of the 26 couples/single individuals who undertook gestational surrogacy, 19 did so with donor eggs. With regard to racial and ethnic background, the majority of parents interviewed identified as white, with the exception of one African American, two Latinos, three Asians, and one of mixed racial background. With the exception of two individuals, all the commissioning parents had attended some college or earned at least a bachelor's degree.

Here I should note how this sample relates to the broader universe of couples who travel to India for surrogacy. Because surrogacy is unregulated, there is very little reliable statistical data on the numbers of couples who travel to India and on the countries from which they originate. Most of the statistics available address numbers of Australian couples traveling to India, and a survey conducted by Surrogacy Australia, a not-for-profit agency, found that in 2012, 200 babies were born via surrogacy in India for Australian couples, compared with 179 in 2011 and 86 in 2010 (Arjunpuri 2013). Another report claims that approximately 250 babies are born each year via surrogacy in India for Australian commissioning parents (with 40 born in Thailand, a growing surrogacy market, and 35 in the United States) (Miller 2013). The actual figures could be even higher, however, as Immigration Department statistics show that the number of babies born to Australian citizens in India jumped from 170 in 2008 to 394 in 2012. While it is difficult to know precisely how many of those children were born via surrogacy, the number of Australians living in India has not risen significantly in the same time period (Whitelaw 2012). Meanwhile, different media reports suggest that approximately half of overseas commissioning parents contracting with Indian surrogates are Australian (Arjunpuri 2013), contradicting reports claiming that Britain sends the highest numbers of people seeking surrogacy services in India, accounting for as many as 1,000 births in India (Bhatia 2012). In a study recently published in the *Journal of Social Welfare and Family Law*, researchers found that increasing numbers of couples from the United Kingdom register children to foreign surrogates (Crawshaw, Blyth, and van den Akker 2012). With respect to U.S. commissioning parents, media reports offer rather vague statements regarding "hundreds of Americans" who travel to India each year for surrogacy (Williams 2013a, 2013b). A report by the Confederation of Indian Industries estimates that around 10,000 foreign couples have visited India so far to commission surrogate pregnancies, and nearly 30 percent of these have been gay or unmarried (Dhillon 2015). Other sources claim that more than 25,000 babies have been born in India as a result of gestational surrogacy; 50 percent of these are from the West (Shetty 2012). Clearly, reliable statistics are hard to come by, and what numbers are available are mainly found in journalistic sources and difficult to verify.

Given the lack of verifiable statistical data, it would be challenging to analyze to what extent my sample reflects the broader universe of individuals seeking surrogacy services in India. However, the available statistics suggest that most commissioning parents travel from Australia, the United Kingdom, and the United States. My sample is not representative of this trend; because I relied partially on introductions through personal networks, my sample includes primarily Western participants, with most of the participants hailing from the United States or Australia.[2] However, the sample is varied enough to reflect the range of experiences of commissioning parents from different countries, and based on my interviews with doctors, I found that this sample nonetheless broadly reflects the population of people traveling to India for ARTs, particularly gestational surrogacy. In 2010, doctors in Mumbai clinics reported that most of their clients seeking surrogacy services came from abroad.

Finally, I should note that my sample reflects a higher proportion of parents who are successful in having children through surrogacy in India. In this study, of the 26 couples/individuals interviewed, 21 had one or more babies through surrogacy in India. However, pregnancy rates with IVF hover around 30 percent. Thus my sample is not representative of the majority of couples who travel to India and are ultimately unsuccessful in their attempts. Rather, this book primarily examines the experiences of the minority of commissioning parents who have successfully reached the goal of a "take-home baby" through gestational surrogacy.

Parents cited a wide range of reasons for pursuing ARTs in India. For many intended parents, traveling to India was only one step in a long history of fertility treatments and miscarriages for infertile couples, or disappointments for gay couples who had sought a child through adoption or foster care. Still others came to India after repeated attempts at surrogacy in other countries, including the United States. I found that motivations for traveling to India depend largely on the country of origin and background of the client. These motivating factors, broadly speaking, include: cost of services, legal constraints (in which commercial surrogacy might be tightly regulated or illegal), availability of services in the home country, and discriminatory practices (in which practitioners deny services to certain groups of people based on age, marital status, or sexual orientation). Of the 39 commissioning parents interviewed in this study, only 9 individuals explicitly mentioned a desire to have a genetically related child as a reason for pursuing surrogacy in India. Instead, the majority of intended parents framed surrogacy as a method of "last resort" for infertile couples who were unable to pursue other strategies for family building, such as adoption.[3]

Surrogates and Egg Donors: In this study, I interviewed 45 Indian women who were surrogate mothers and/or egg donors, including 6 agents. I was able to speak with many of these women several times during the course of their experiences with surrogacy. I also gathered observations from women who were at distinct points in the process of surrogacy: I interviewed 8 women who were in the preparatory stages for embryo transfer, 18 who were pregnant at some point during my fieldwork, 11 who were former surrogates, and 4 who underwent embryo transfer but did not become pregnant. I also interviewed 4 women who were egg donors and/or agents only. Women's encounters with ARTs indicated the varied ways in which they become entrenched in the industry; often, women held simultaneous positions as surrogate or egg donor and agent. That is, participation in one area (surrogacy, egg donation, or agent work) often led to further work in another area.

Women came from primarily low-income families and most pursued surrogacy as a solution to their financial hardships such as debts or lack of housing. The majority of the women were married, with the exception of three widows, two divorced women, and one unmarried woman. All the women had previously given birth, with the exception of one childless woman. Women completed varying levels of education, from primary school to high school. Nearly all the women identified as housewives, and those who worked outside the home typically did domestic work, factory work, or work in the garment industry. With regard to religious background, most participants identified as Hindu or Buddhist, with several women identifying as Christian or Muslim.

Caste remains a sensitive issue in India and I followed my translator's cues as to whether and when it was appropriate to discuss it. In most cases, it was considered an inappropriate and sensitive topic, so we did not include caste in our list of background questions for women. Religion, however, was a somewhat less sensitive question than caste, so I was able to discern to some degree women's caste and class background through their religious background, particularly for women who identified as Buddhist converts. Many of these families continued to practice Hindu rituals and they often identified as "Hindu Buddhist," and I noted that some women had framed photos of Dr. B. R. Ambedkar in their homes, indicating Dalit, or low-caste status women.[4] As one of my translators informed me, these are clear signs of caste and class background. Though only 15 out of 45 women (around 30 percent) identified as Buddhist (suggesting Dalit status), several of my translators believed that the proportion of Dalit women in this study was significantly higher. While most foreign clients expressed no preference regarding caste in egg donation or surrogacy, caste remains an implicit organizing criterion within assisted reproduction in India. Indeed, Indian consumers of ARTs frequently take into account caste background in their decisions regarding gamete donation and surrogacy (Tewary 2012; Rai 2010).

When asked their reasons for wanting to become a surrogate or egg donor, all the women reported financial need as their primary motivation. In general, the women commented that they needed funds to pay for their children's education, housing, debts, or their daughter's marriage (indicating that the practice of dowry, though illegal, continues to exist). However, it is important to note that while all cited their need for income, the women represented a diversity of class backgrounds. They came from mostly working class and middle class families, with few in dire poverty. My visits to their homes confirmed the diverse class backgrounds of women in my study, as I noted the wide differences in housing and living arrangements.

Doctors: I interviewed a total of 21 doctors in 16 clinics over the course of my research, including: 17 doctors representing 14 clinics in Mumbai, 2 doctors in 1 clinic in Anand, and 2 doctors in 1 clinic in Delhi. While I conducted many first-time and follow-up interviews with these doctors throughout my research, I carried out more focused research with doctors in 4 Mumbai clinics in 2010. All but one of the doctors spoke fluent English and most had received some medical training abroad, either in the United Kingdom or the United States. Of these doctors, ten were male and eleven were female, representing a fairly even gender balance. The doctors in this study represent a range of specialties and include reproductive endocrinologists, psychologists, obstetricians, gynecologists, and occupational health physicians.

As with other aspects of assisted reproduction in India, there is no systematic data available on clinical practices or the number of clinics throughout the country. The Indian Society for Assisted Reproduction (ISAR) boasts more than 600 members, and there are over 350 member

IVF clinics in India with several centers dedicated to commercial surrogacy. However, not all operating clinics are ISAR members, and Dr. R. S. Sharma of the ICMR estimates that there are 700 to 800 IVF clinics across the country (Outlook India 2009), while the National Commission for Women, on the other hand, suggests that approximately 3,000 clinics are in operation (Kannan 2009). Within this context, it is difficult to situate the clinics in which I conducted research. However, while many IVF clinics cater to the Indian and nonresident Indian (NRI) population, the clinics in my sample that offered surrogacy services attracted primarily foreign clients. One doctor I interviewed estimated that approximately 80 percent of her surrogacy clients traveled from abroad, while another estimated he received around 15 to 20 couples per month, primarily from abroad. Indeed, all the doctors in this study who offered surrogacy services indicated that most of their surrogacy clients came from abroad (while IVF clients tended to be Indian). Moreover, as mentioned above, the doctors in these clinics welcomed gay clients (while others refused services to same-sex couples), thus affecting the sample of commissioning parents in this study.

Other Actors: Finally, there were a number of people whom I interviewed that occupy an important role in the surrogacy industry in India. These include traveling egg donors from South Africa, ART legal experts, medical tourism agents and brokers, and American adjudicators involved in processing citizenship requests for babies born outside the United States.

NOTES

INTRODUCTION

1 All personal names in this book are pseudonyms. I have replaced participants' names with other names of the appropriate gender and place of origin, depending on the participant's background. I have also replaced names of places and institutions such as clinics and hospitals.

2 "Nadipur" is a pseudonym for the city in which the majority of the surrogates I interviewed, including Nishi, lived. It is part of the Mumbai Metropolitan Region, which has a population of more than 18 million and includes the cities of Ambernath, Badlapur, Kalyan-Dombivali, Mira-Bhayander, Mumbai, Navi Mumbai, Thane, and Ulhasnagar. According to the 2011 Census, Nadipur had a population of more than 500,000, with males comprising 53 percent of the population and females 47 percent. Nadipur is an industrial area, known as a hub of the garment industry in which many Western clothing brands are copied. The city is reachable by road or by Mumbai's suburban railway system, which is how my assistants and I would travel to conduct interviews. From central Mumbai, the train journey takes approximately one and a half hours.

3 All estimates of fees, payments, or money exchanged are based on the 2010 average exchange rate of 1 U.S. dollar to 45.68 Indian rupees.

4 While there are few ethnographic studies that examine processes of racialization in the context of transnational surrogacy, scholars in gender studies and philosophy have begun to focus explicitly on race in studies of surrogacy (see Harrison 2014; Banerjee 2014).

5 While there is a shift toward nuclear family living arrangements, particularly in urban areas, some families continue to live in extended family arrangements together with the husband's parents.

CHAPTER 1. PUBLIC HEALTH AND ASSISTED REPRODUCTION IN INDIA

1 A report by the Confederation of Indian Industry estimates that the surrogacy industry generates $2.3 billion annually (Gupta 2011). This figure is widely cited in media and research articles, while others note the industry is worth $445 million (IANS 2008). Current data on the surrogacy industry in India, however, are difficult to obtain and often unavailable, contributing to what Anindita Majumdar calls its "mythic value" on the global market for reproductive services (2014, 220).

2 In comparison, in 2002 in the United States, 68 percent of mothers who had live births received an ultrasound, while 99 percent of births were delivered in hospitals (Martin et al. 2003).

3 Due to the lack of regulation, it is difficult to find reliable statistics regarding the numbers of births or numbers of clients who travel to India for surrogacy services; *Time* magazine claims that 25,000 couples travel to India each year (Bhowmick 2013), while the *Telegraph* estimates that 2,000 surrogacy births occurred in India in 2011 (Bhatia 2012). While it is difficult to assess these estimates, the low rates of success with IVF contextualize their large discrepancy. In 2009 the Indian Society for Assisted Reproduction (ISAR) conducted an estimated 18,000 IVF cycles (their statistics do not say how many couples these cycles served or how many were foreign), averaging a 30 percent rate of pregnancy. The group says that only half of the clinics throughout India are members, making the total number of IVF cycles sought much higher (Rai 2010). Nonmembers may have lower success rates. As a result, the number of clients traveling for surrogacy should be significantly higher than the number of surrogacy births—although tenfold seems unlikely.

4 In contrast, many countries, including China, the Czech Republic, Denmark, France, Germany, Italy, Spain, Sweden, Turkey, and some U.S. states ban surrogacy altogether. Other countries have imposed partial bans, such as Australia (Victoria), Brazil, Hong Kong, Hungary, Israel, South Africa, and the United Kingdom. Among these countries, Canada, Greece, South Africa, Israel, and the United Kingdom permit surrogacy, though it is subject to governmental regulations. There are still other countries with no regulations at all, including Belgium, Finland, India, and some U.S. states (Teman 2010). While surrogacy surged in India in the first decade of the twenty-first century, commercial surrogacy remained most prevalent in the state of California and Israel—where the state restricts surrogacy to Jewish citizens. Indian surrogacy practices closely mirror the liberal market model of surrogacy in California, where private, commercial agencies manage surrogacy arrangements. These agencies rely on their own criteria for screening, matching, and regulating surrogacy agreements, and in India clinics operate largely without state intervention. They also benefit from government support for medical tourism.

5 ICMR guidelines dictate that surrogates cannot have more than five live births (including surrogate births), yet they must also have had at least one child of their own to prove fertility. The argument is that if a woman has given birth to children of her own, she will be less likely to bond emotionally with a child to whom she is not genetically related. At the same time, studies indicate that with each subsequent live birth a woman experiences, she will be at greater risk of experiencing complications during pregnancy and childbirth. Note that between the 2008 and 2010 Drafts, the ICMR raised the upper limit of pregnancies for surrogates from three to five.

CHAPTER 2. MAKING KINSHIP, OTHERING WOMEN

1 See Surrogacy India, http://www.surrogacyindia.com/About-SurrogacyIndia. html, accessed February 17, 2015.

2 See https://sites.google.com/a/surrogacyindia.com/enrollment/si-program/si-brochure/Flyers.pdf?attredirects=0&d=1, accessed February 23, 2015.

3 See Howell (2006) for discussion of "kinning" practices among unrelated family members in the context of transnational adoption.

4 In her essay, "Can the Subaltern Speak?" Gayatri Spivak (1988) unravels the ways in which a particular script of rescue, that of "white men saving brown women from brown men," was vital to the operation of British colonialism. Leila Ahmed (1993) too illuminates the ways in which British colonial authorities in Egypt relied on the rhetoric of women's emancipation for their colonial mission. In doing so, Western feminism came to serve as a "handmaiden" to colonialism. As these scholars demonstrate, political imperial projects relied on the elaboration of rescue narratives in their "civilizing missions," with women's emancipation acting as the mobilizing rationale.

CHAPTER 3. EGG DONATION AND EXOTIC BEAUTY

1 In general, parents who wished to purchase eggs from a white woman paid approximately U.S.$10–11,000, while eggs from an Indian woman cost around U.S.$700.

2 See, for example, Alvarez (2004); Ikemoto (2009); and Weiss (2001).

3 It is worth noting that sperm donation is rare in the context of surrogacy. In my study there were no cases in which sperm donation was necessary; typically, the husband/male partner provided the sperm that would fertilize the donor egg through IVF. In the case of gay male couples, the couple would negotiate which partner would provide the genetic material; I encountered several cases in which both partners opted to become genetic parents through IVF with one egg donor and two surrogates.

4 Dr. Guha's use of the term "Oriental" may reflect the influence of British English in Indian speech, where the term may not be considered particularly offensive and is generally used to refer to people from East and Southeast Asia. He was the only doctor to use the term. Other doctors I interviewed used racial categories such as "Asian" to refer to people of Asian descent. It is perhaps worth noting that Dr. Guha was one of the few doctors I interviewed who had not received any medical training outside India. All the other doctors were educated abroad, reflecting perhaps a cosmopolitan understanding of the various racial categories used in different contexts.

CHAPTER 4. THE MAKING OF CITIZENS AND PARENTS

1 See, for example, *India Today* 2009; *Times of India* 2012a, 2012b; Mahapatra 2008; Roy 2010b; Roy 2011.

2 One such case involves Kari Ann Volden, a single Norwegian woman who commissioned a surrogate pregnancy in India with eggs from an Indian woman and sperm from a Danish man. The surrogate gave birth to twin boys who were considered "stateless" and unable to leave India for the first fifteen months of their lives, as the Norwegian government did not consider Volden their mother (and consequently the boys could not obtain Norwegian citizenship) and the Indian government did not consider them Indian. See Kr.løkke (2012) for an extended discussion of this case.

CHAPTER 6. MEDICALIZED BIRTH AND THE CONSTRUCTION OF RISK

1 In 2012, the most recent year for which preliminary data are available, 32.8 percent of 3,952,937 births in the United States were cesarean deliveries. See Hamilton et al. 2013.

CHAPTER 7. CONSTRAINED AGENCY AND POWER IN SURROGATES' EVERYDAY LIVES

1 See Pande (2014c) for discussion of broker/surrogate relationships in another surrogacy clinic in India.

2 For examples of ethnographic research that examine forms of resistance and agency within the context of social, economic, and institutional inequalities, see Brennan (2004); Constable (1997, 2009b); Kempadoo (2005); and Parreñas (2008).

3 Media coverage on surrogacy in India and around the globe routinely underscores the relationship between poverty and surrogacy, fostering the notion that contract pregnancy offers poor women the opportunity of a lifetime. In the *Times of India*, Bella Jaisinghani (2010) reported that "a reed-thin Nafisa" and her child were "the picture of poverty, skin stretched taut over bones, for they were barely able to fill their stomachs on most days." Jaisinghani went on to write, "Desperate for that one push that'll take them out of the hard life, it is the poorest of the poor, the slum dwellers of Mumbai, who are renting their wombs and sustaining commercial surrogacy in the city." In *Der Spiegel Online*, Sandra Schulz wrote that Suman Dodia, for example, would earn U.S.$4,500 for carrying a British couple's child, a sum that would have taken her fifteen years to earn as a maid (Schulz 2008). Abigail Haworth, reporting for *Marie Claire*, told the story of Sofia Vohra, a surrogate who previously earned U.S.$25 a month as a glass-crusher; Vohra said, "This is not exploitation. Crushing glass for fifteen hours a day is exploitation. The baby's parents have given me a chance to make good marriages for my daughters. That's a big weight off my mind" (Haworth 2007). These representations of surrogates' stories highlight opportunity, choice, and fair exchange, yet they do not present the complete picture of Indian surrogacy and fail to address the ways in which gender, race, ethnicity, caste, and class mediate women's expectations and beliefs about surrogacy. For additional examples, see Desai (2012); Gentleman (2008); and Warner (2008).

4 In recent years, there has been an increase in student enrollment in English-medium schools and a drop in students opting for Marathi-medium schools in Mumbai (Chavan 2011). Yet among the working-class women in this study, access to English-language instruction was extremely limited due to the costs of education, making Nishi's knowledge of English even more remarkable. Nishi herself wanted to send her daughters to English-medium schools but regretted that she could not afford the cost.

5 Among the eligibility requirements for women who wished to become surrogates, doctors required that married women have the permission of their husbands.

6 Since Antara's surrogacy experience, payment for gestational surrogates in 2010 increased to U.S.$4,000–6,000 for most of the surrogates included in this study, depending on the clinic they attended.

7 See Dumont (1980 [1970]); and Marriott (1976).

CONCLUSION

1 See Hamdy (2012) for a discussion of practice-oriented approaches to bioethics in the context of organ transplantation in Egypt.

APPENDIX

1 I interviewed intended parents under a variety of circumstances: in some instances I interviewed couples together, while in others I interviewed only one member of a couple. With the exception of two single males, all the intended parents were either married or in a live-in, committed relationship.

2 Rather than focus on a single nationality, I aimed to recruit commissioning parents from a diversity of countries and nationalities in order to illustrate the range of motivations and experiences of individuals seeking ARTs in India.

3 The reasons for rejecting adoption as an option varied, depending on the home country of the intended parents. Typically these couples claimed they were unable to pursue adoption for various reasons, including medical histories that precluded them from being selected as "fit" parents; advanced age; a decreasing number of domestic adoptions available in the home country; discrimination against same-sex couples; and the long waits and bureaucratic processes associated with international adoption.

4 Dr. B. R. Ambedkar, a leader of the Dalit movement, called for the conversion of Dalits to Buddhism as an act of rejection of the caste-based system that relegated them to the lowest rungs of the hierarchy.

BIBLIOGRAPHY

ACOG. 2005. "Perinatal Risks Associated with Assisted Reproductive Technology: ACOG Committee Opinion No. 324." *Obstetrics & Gynecology* 106:1143–1146.

ACRJ. 2005. "A New Vision for Advancing Our Movement for Reproductive Health, Reproductive Rights and Reproductive Justice." http://forwardtogether.org/assets/docs/ACRJ-A-New-Vision.pdf.

Agigian, Amy. 2004. *Baby Steps: How Lesbian Alternative Insemination Is Changing the World.* Middletown: Wesleyan University Press.

Ahearn, Laura M. 2001. *Invitations to Love: Literacy, Love Letters, and Social Change in Nepal.* Ann Arbor: University of Michigan Press.

Ahluwalia, Sanjam. 2008. *Reproductive Restraints: Birth Control in India, 1877–1947.* Urbana: University of Illinois Press.

Ahmed, Leila. 1993. *Women and Gender in Islam: Historical Roots of a Modern Debate.* New Haven: Yale University Press.

Almeling, Rene. 2011. *Sex Cells: The Medical Market for Eggs and Sperm.* Berkeley: University of California Press.

Alonso, Ana María. 1994. "The Politics of Space, Time and Substance: State Formation, Nationalism, and Ethnicity." *Annual Review of Anthropology* 23:379–405.

Althusser, Louis. 1971. "Ideology and Ideological State Apparatus (Notes Towards an Investigation)." In *Lenin and Philosophy and Other Essays*, edited by Louis Althusser, 127–186. London: New Left Books.

Alvarez, Lizette. 2004. "Spreading Scandinavian Genes without Viking Boats." *New York Times*, September 30.

Amrith, Sunil. 2009. *Health in India since Independence.* Manchester: Brooks World Poverty Institute.

Anagnost, Ann. 2000. "Scenes of Misrecognition: Maternal Citizenship in the Age of Transnational Adoption." *positions* 8 (2):389–421.

Anand Kumar, T. C. 2003. "Advent of Medically Assisted Reproductive Technologies (MART) in India." In *The Art and Science of Assisted Reproductive Techniques*, edited by Gautam N. Allahbadia, Rita Basuray Das, and Rubina Merchant, 3–7. New Delhi: Taylor & Francis Group.

Anderson, Benedict. 1983. *Imagined Communities: Reflections on the Origin and Spread of Nationalism.* London: Verso.

Appadurai, Arjun. 1996. *Modernity at Large: Cultural Dimensions of Globalization.* Minneapolis: University of Minnesota Press.

Aravamudan, Gita. 2015. Regulate, Don't Eliminate. *Hindu*, http://www.thehindu.com/opinion/op-ed/ban-on-commercial-surrogacy-regulate-dont-eliminate/article7842740.ece.

Arjunpuri, Chaitra. 2013. "India's Growing 'Rent-a-Womb' Industry." *Al Jazeera*, http://www.aljazeera.com/indepth/features/2013/01/2013128122419799224.html?utm_content=automate&utm_campaign=Trial6&utm_source=NewSocialFlow&utm_term=plustweets&utm_medium=MasterAccount.

Arms, Suzanne. 1975. *Immaculate Deception: A New Look at Women and Childbirth in America*. Boston: Houghton Mifflin.

Arnold, David. 1993. *Colonizing the Body: State Medicine and Epidemic Disease in Nineteenth-Century India*. Berkeley: University of California Press.

——. 2006. "Official Attitudes to Population, Birth Control and Reproductive Health in India, 1921–1946." In *Reproductive Health in India: History, Politics, Controversies*, edited by Sarah Hodges, 22–50. New Delhi: Orient Longman.

Baber, Zaheer. 2004. "'Race,' Religion and Riots: The 'Racialization' of Communal Identity and Conflict in India." *Sociology* 38 (4):701–718. doi: 10.1177/0038038504045860.

——. 2010. "Racism without Races: Reflections on Racialization and Racial Projects." *Sociology Compass* 4 (4):241–248.

Bailey, Alison. 2011. "Reconceiving Surrogacy: Toward a Reproductive Justice Account of Indian Surrogacy." *Hypatia* 26 (4):715–741.

Balibar, Étienne. 1991. "Racism and Nationalism." In *Race, Nation and Class: Ambiguous Identities*, edited by Étienne Balibar and Immanuel Wallerstein, 37–67. London: Verso.

Banerjee, Amrita. 2010. "Reorienting the Ethics of Transnational Surrogacy as a Feminist Pragmatist." *Pluralist* 5 (3):107–127.

——. 2014. "Race and a Transnational Reproductive Caste System: Indian Transnational Surrogacy." *Hypatia* 29 (1):113–128.

Banerji, Debabar. 2001. "Landmarks in the Development of Health Services in India." In *Public Health and the Poverty of Reforms*, edited by Imrana Qadeer, Kasturi Sen, and K. R. Nayar, 39–50. New Delhi: Sage.

——. 2004. "The People and Health Service Development in India: A Brief Overview." *International Journal of Health Services* 34 (1):123–142.

Banton, Michael. 1977. *The Idea of Race*. London: Tavistock.

Barrett, Jon F. R., Mary E. Hannah, Eileen K. Hutton, Andrew R. Willan, Alexander C. Allen, B. Anthony Armson, Amiram Gafni, K. S. Joseph, Dalah Mason, Arne Ohlsson, Susan Ross, J. Johanna Sanchez, and Elizabeth V. Asztalos. 2013. "A Randomized Trial of Planned Cesarean or Vaginal Delivery for Twin Pregnancy." *New England Journal of Medicine* 369 (14):1295–1305. doi: doi:10.1056/NEJMoa1214939.

Baru, Rama V. 1998. *Private Health Care in India: Social Characteristics and Trends*. New Delhi: Sage.

Basu, Srimati. 2015. *The Trouble with Marriage: Feminists Confront Law and Violence in India*. Berkeley: University of California Press.

Becker, Gay. 2000. *The Elusive Embryo: How Women and Men Approach New Reproductive Technologies*. Berkeley: University of California Press.

Becker, Gay, Anneliese Butler, and Robert D. Nachtigall. 2005. "Resemblance Talk: A Challenge for Parents Whose Children Were Conceived with Donor Gametes in the U.S." *Social Science & Medicine* 61 (6):1300–1309. doi: 10.1016/j. socscimed.2005.01.018.

Beeson, Diane, Marcy Darnovsky, and Abby Lippman. 2015. "What's in a Name? Variations in Terminology of Third-Party Reproduction." *Reproductive BioMedicine Online* 31 (6): 805–814.

Belizán, José M., Fernando Althabe, Fernando C Barros, Sophie Alexander, Elaine Showalter, Anne Griffin, Arachu Castro, and Hilda Bastian. 1999. "Rates and Implications of Caesarean Sections in Latin America: Ecological Study." *British Medical Journal* 319 (7222):1397–1402.

Beteille, Andre. 2001. "Race and Caste." *Hindu*, March 10. http://www.thehindu.com/thehindu/2001/03/10/stories/05102523.htm.

Bharadwaj, Aditya. 2000. "How Some Indian Baby Makers Are Made: Media Narratives and Assisted Conception in India." *Anthropology & Medicine* 7 (1):63–78.

———. 2002. "Conception Politics: Medical Egos, Media Spotlights, and the Contest over Test Tube Firsts in India." In *Infertility around the Globe: New Thinking on Childlessness, Gender, and Reproductive Technologies*, edited by Marcia Inhorn and Frank Van Balen, 315–333. Berkeley: University of California Press.

———. 2003. "Why Adoption Is Not an Option in India: The Visibility of Infertility, the Secrecy of Donor Insemination, and Other Cultural Complexities." *Social Science and Medicine* 56 (9):1867–1880.

———. 2006. "Sacred Conceptions: Clinical Theodicies, Uncertain Science, and Technologies of Procreation in India." *Culture, Medicine and Psychiatry* 30 (4):451–465.

Bhatia, Shekhar. 2012. "Revealed: How More and More Britons Are Paying Indian Women to Become Surrogate Mothers." *Telegraph*, http://www.telegraph.co.uk/health/healthnews/9292343/Revealed-how-and-more-Britons-are-paying-Indian-women-to-become-surrogate-mothers.html.

Bhowmick, Nilanjana. 2013. "Why People Are Angry about India's New Surrogacy Rules." *Time*, http://world.time.com/2013/02/15/why-people-are-angry-about-indias-new-surrogacy-laws/.

Blyth, Eric, Petra Thorn, and Tewes Wischmann. 2011. "CBRC and Psychosocial Counselling: Assessing Needs and Developing an Ethical Framework for Practice." *Reproductive BioMedicine Online* 23 (5):642–651. doi: 10.1016/j.rbmo.2011.07.009.

Boehm, F. H., and C. R. Graves. 1994. "Caesarean Birth." In *Manual of Clinical Problems in Obstetrics and Gynecology*, edited by M. E. Rivlin and R. W. Martin, 158–162. Boston: Little Brown.

Boris, Eileen, and Rhacel Salazar Parreñas. 2010. *Intimate Labors: Cultures, Technologies, and the Politics of Care*. Stanford: Stanford University Press.

Brennan, Denise. 2004. *What's Love Got to Do with It? Transnational Desires and Sex Tourism in the Dominican Republic*. Durham: Duke University Press.

Bridges, Khiara M. 2011. *Reproducing Race: An Ethnography of Pregnancy as a Site of Racialization*. Berkeley: University of California Press.

Brochmann, Grete, and Idunn Seland. 2010. "Citizenship Policies and Ideas of Nation-hood in Scandinavia." *Citizenship Studies* 14 (4):429–443.

Brodwin, Paul. 2002. "Genetics, Identity, and the Anthropology of Essentialism." *Anthropological Quarterly* 75 (2):323–330.

Brooks, A. A., M. R. Johnson, P. J. Steer, M. E. Pawson, and H. I. Abdalla. 1995. "Birth Weight: Nature or Nurture?" *Early Human Development* 42 (1):29–35.

Browner, Carole H., and Nancy Ann Press. 1995. "The Normalization of Prenatal Diagnostic Screening." In *Conceiving the New World Order: The Global Politics of Reproduction*, edited by Faye Ginsburg and Rayna Rapp, 307–322. Berkeley: University of California Press.

Butler, Judith. 1997. *The Psychic Life of Power: Theories in Subjection*. Stanford: Stanford University Press.

Buzinde, Christine N., and Careen Yarnal. 2012. "Therapeutic Landscapes and Post-colonial Theory: A Theoretical Approach to Medical Tourism." *Social Science & Medicine* 74 (5):783–787. doi: http://dx.doi.org/10.1016/j.socscimed.2011.11.016.

Campbell, Ben. 2007. "Racialization, Genes and the Reinventions of Nation in Europe." In *Race, Ethnicity and Nation: Perspectives from Kinship and Genetics*, edited by Peter Wade, 95–124. New York: Berghahn Books.

Carsten, Janet. 2000. *Cultures of Relatedness: New Approaches to the Study of Kinship*. Cambridge: Cambridge University Press.

——. 2001. "Substantivism, Antisubstantivism, and Anti-Antisubstantivism." In *Relative Values: Reconfiguring Kinship Studies*, edited by Sarah Franklin and Susan McKinnon, 29–53. Durham: Duke University Press.

——. 2004. *After Kinship*. Cambridge: Cambridge University Press.

Casper, Monica J. 2011. "Reproductive Tourism." *Feminist Wire*, http://thefeministwire.com/2011/04/reproductive-tourism/.

Chakrabarty, Dipesh. 1994. "Modernity and Ethnicity in India." *South Asia: Journal of South Asian Studies* 17 (s1):143–155.

Chatterjee, Nilanjana, and Nancy E. Riley. 2001. "Planning an Indian Modernity: The Gendered Politics of Fertility Control." *Signs* 26 (3):811–845.

Chatterjee, Partha. 1989a. "Colonialism, Nationalism, and Colonialized Women: The Contest in India." *American Ethnologist* 16 (4):622–633.

——. 1989b. "The Nationalist Resolution of the Women's Question." In *Recasting Women: Essays in Indian Colonial History*, edited by Kumkum Sangari and Sudesh Vaid, 233–253. New Brunswick: Rutgers University Press.

Chavan, Prajakta. 2011. "Students Prefer English Medium to Studying in Other Languages." *Hindustan Times*, http://www.hindustantimes.com/India-news/Mumbai/Students-prefer-English-medium-to-studying-in-other-languages/Article1-761222.aspx.

Chinai, Rupa, and Rahul Goswami. 2007. "Medical Visas Mark Growth of Indian Medical Tourism." *Bulletin of the World Health Organization* 85 (3):164–165.

Chu, Henry. 2006. "Wombs for Rent, Cheap." *Los Angeles Times*, April 19, http://articles.latimes.com/2006/apr/19/world/fg-surrogate19.

Clement, Sarah. 2001. "Psychological Aspects of Caesarean Section." *Best Practice & Research Clinical Obstetrics & Gynaecology* 15 (1):109–126.

Coffey, Diane. 2015. "Prepregnancy Body Mass and Weight Gain during Pregnancy in India and Sub-Saharan Africa." *Proceedings of the National Academy of Sciences.* doi: 10.1073/pnas.1416964112.

Cohen, Lawrence. 2005. "Operability, Bioavailability, and Exception." In *Global Assemblages: Technology, Politics, and Ethics as Anthropological Problems*, edited by Aihwa Ong and Stephen Collier. Oxford: Blackwell Publishing.

Cohen, Nancy Wainer, and Lois J Estner. 1983. *Silent Knife: Cesarean Prevention and Vaginal Birth after Cesarean*. South Hadley, Mass.: Bergin & Garvey.

Colen, Shellee. 1995. "'Like a Mother to Them': Stratified Reproduction and West Indian Childcare Workers and Employers in New York." In *Conceiving the New World Order*, edited by Faye Ginsburg and Rayna Rapp, 78–102. Berkeley: University of California Press.

Constable, Nicole. 1997. *Maid to Order in Hong Kong: Stories of Filipina Workers.* Ithaca: Cornell University Press.

———. 2009a. "The Commodification of Intimacy: Marriage, Sex, and Reproductive Labor." *Annual Review of Anthropology* 38:49–64.

———. 2009b. "Migrant Workers and the Many States of Protest in Hong Kong." *Critical Asian Studies* 41:143–164.

Cook, Michael. 2012. "17-Year-Old Indian Girl Dies after Egg Donation." *BioEdge*, http://www.bioedge.org/bioethics/bioethics_article/10157.

Cooper, Melinda, and Catherine Waldby. 2014. *Clinical Labor: Tissue Donors and Research Subjects in the Global Bioeconomy*. Durham: Duke University Press.

Corea, Gena. 1985. *The Mother Machine: Reproductive Technologies from Artificial Insemination to Artificial Wombs*. 1st ed. New York: Harper & Row.

Crawshaw, Marilyn, Eric Blyth, and Olga van den Akker. 2012. "The Changing Profile of Surrogacy in the U.K.: Implications for National and International Policy and Practice." *Journal of Social Welfare and Family Law* 34 (3):267–277. doi: 10.1080/09649069.2012.750478.

Crooks, V. A., L. Turner, J. Snyder, R. Johnston, and P. Kingsbury. 2011. "Promoting Medical Tourism to India: Messages, Images, and the Marketing of International Patient Travel." *Social Science & Medicine* 72 (5):726–732.

Cussins, Charis. 1998. "'Quit Sniveling, Cryo-Baby. We'll Work Out Which One's Your Mama!'" In *Cyborg Babies: From Techno-Sex to Techno-Tots*, edited by Robbie Davis-Floyd and Joseph Dumit, 40–66. New York: Routledge.

Daniels, Cynthia R., and Erin Heidt-Forsythe. 2012. "Gendered Eugenics and the Problematic of Free Market Reproductive Technologies: Sperm and Egg Donation in the United States." *Signs* 37 (3):719–747. doi: 10.1086/662964.

Das, Purba. 2014. "'Is Caste Race?' Discourses of Racial Indianization." *Journal of Intercultural Communication Research* 43 (3):264–282. doi: 10.1080/17475759.2014.944556.

DasGupta, Sayantani, and Shamita Das Dasgupta. 2010. "Motherhood Jeopardized: Reproductive Technologies in Indian Communities." In *The Globalization of Moth-

erhood: Deconstructions and Reconstructions of Biology and Care, edited by Wendy Chavkin and JaneMaree Maher, 131–153. New York: Routledge.

———. 2014a. *Globalization and Transnational Surrogacy in India: Outsourcing Life.* Lanham, Mass.: Lexington Books.

———. 2014b. "Shifting Sands: Transnational Surrogacy, E-Motherhood, and Nation Building." In *Globalization and Transnational Surrogacy in India: Outsourcing Life*, edited by Sayantani DasGupta and Shamita Das Dasgupta, 67–77. Lanham, Mass.: Lexington Books.

David, Richard, and James Collins Jr. 2007. "Disparities in Infant Mortality: What's Genetics Got to Do with It?" *American Journal of Public Health* 97 (7):1191–1197.

Davis, Dana-Ain. 2009. "The Politics of Reproduction: The Troubling Case of Nadya Suleman and Assisted Reproductive Technology." *Transforming Anthropology* 17 (2):105–116.

Davis, Mike. 2001. *Late Victorian Holocausts: El Niño Famines and the Making of the Third World.* London: Verso.

De Sam Lazaro, Fred. 2011. "India's New Baby Boom." *PBS*, http://www.pbs.org/newshour/rundown/2011/08/reporters-notebook-indias-new-baby-boom.html.

Deomampo, Daisy. 2013. "Gendered Geographies of Reproductive Tourism." *Gender & Society* 27 (4):514–537.

Desai, Kishwar. 2012. "India's Surrogate Mothers Are Risking Their Lives. They Urgently Need Protection." *Guardian*, http://www.guardian.co.uk/commentisfree/2012/jun/05/india-surrogates-impoverished-die?fb=optOut.

Deshpande, Ashwini. 2005. "Affirmative Action in India and the United States." In *Equity and Development.* Washington, D.C.: World Bank.

Dhillon, Amrit. 2015. "India to Introduce Law Requiring Bond for Surrogacy Hopefuls." *Sydney Morning Herald*, http://www.smh.com.au/world/india-to-introduce-law-requiring-bond-for-surrogacy-hopefuls-20150626-ghybq9.html.

Dikötter, Frank. 1997. "Racial Discourse in China: Continuities and Permutations." In *The Construction of Racial Identities in China and Japan: Historical and Contemporary Perspectives*, edited by Frank Dikötter, 12–33. Honolulu: University of Hawai'i Press.

Dorow, Sara. 2006. "Racialized Choices: Chinese Adoption and the 'White Noise' of Blackness." *Critical Sociology* 32 (2–3):357–379. doi: 10.1163/156916306777835277.

Duggal, Ravi, and Sucheta Amin. 1989. "Costs of Health Care: A Household Survey in an Indian District." Mumbai: Foundation for Research in Community Health.

Dumont, Louis. 1980 [1970]. *Homo Hierarchicus: The Caste System and Its Implications.* Chicago: University of Chicago Press.

Eastman, Nicholson J. 1932. "The Role of Frontier America in the Development of Cesarean Section." *American Journal of Obstetrics and Gynecology* 24:919–929.

Edwards, Jeanette. 1993. "Explicit Connections: Ethnographic Enquiry in Northwest England." In *Technologies of Procreation: Kinship in the Age of Assisted Conception*, edited by Jeanette Edwards, Sarah Franklin, Eric Hirsch, Frances Price, and Marilyn Strathern, 61–86. Manchester: Manchester University Press.

Eng, David L. 2003. "Transnational Adoption and Queer Diasporas." *Social Text* 21 (3):1–37.

Ergas, Yasmine. 2013. "Babies without Borders: Human Rights, Human Dignity and the Regulation of International Commercial Surrogacy." *Emory International Law Review*: 1–69.

Fixmer-Oraiz, Natalie. 2013. "Speaking of Solidarity: Transnational Gestational Surrogacy and the Rhetorics of Reproductive (In)Justice." *Frontiers: A Journal of Women Studies* 34 (3):126–163.

Frank, Zippi Brand, dir. 2009. *Google Baby*. Alexandria: Filmmakers Library.

Franklin, Sarah. 2013. *Biological Relatives: IVF, Stem Cells, and the Future of Kinship*. Durham: Duke University Press.

Franklin, Sarah, and Helena Ragoné. 1998. *Reproducing Reproduction: Kinship, Power, and Technological Innovation*. Philadelphia: University of Pennsylvania Press.

Fruzzetti, Lina, and Ákos Östör. 1984. *Kinship and Ritual in Bengal: Anthropological Essays*. New Delhi: South Asia Books.

Fuller, Thomas. 2014. "Thailand's Business in Paid Surrogates May Be Foundering in a Moral Quagmire." *New York Times*, http://nyti.ms/1ARtUrA.

Gailey, Christine Ward. 1996. "Politics, Colonialism, and the Mutable Color of Pacific Islanders." In *Race and Other Misadventures: Essays in Honor of Ashley Montagu in His Ninetieth Year*, edited by Larry T. Reynolds and Leonard Lieberman, 36–49. New York: General Hall.

———. 2010. *Blue-Ribbon Babies and Labors of Love: Race, Class and Gender in U.S. Adoption Practice*. Austin: University of Texas Press.

Garcia, Richard. 2003. "The Misuse of Race in Medical Diagnosis." *Chronicle of Higher Education* 49:B15.

Gentleman, Amelia. 2008. "India Nurtures Business of Surrogate Motherhood." *New York Times*, May 10.

Gesler, Wilbert M. 1992. "Therapeutic Landscapes: Medical Issues in Light of the New Cultural Geography." *Social Science & Medicine* 34 (7):735–746.

Ghosh, Sancheetha, and K. S. James. 2010. "Levels and Trends in Caesarean Births: Cause for Concern?" *Economic & Political Weekly* 45 (5):19–22.

Gilroy, Paul. 1987. *"There Ain't No Black in the Union Jack": The Cultural Politics of Race and Nation*. London: Hutchinson.

Ginsburg, Faye, and Rayna Rapp. 1995. *Conceiving the New World Order: The Global Politics of Reproduction*. Berkeley: University of California Press.

Glenn, Evelyn Nakano. 2002. *Unequal Freedom: How Race and Gender Shaped American Citizenship and Labor*. Cambridge: Harvard University Press.

Gould, Stephen Jay. 1981. *The Mismeasure of Man*. New York: Norton.

Greenhalgh, Susan. 2008. *Just One Child: Science and Policy in Deng's China*. Berkeley: University of California Press.

Gupta, Akhil, and James Ferguson. 1992. "Beyond 'Culture': Space, Identity, and the Politics of Difference." *Cultural Anthropology* 7 (1):6–23. doi: 10.1525/can.1992.7.1.02a00020.

———. 1997. "Discipline and Practice: 'The Field' as Site, Method, and Location in Anthropology." In *Anthropological Locations: Boundaries and Grounds of a Field Science*, edited by Akhil Gupta and James Ferguson, 1–46. Berkeley: University of California Press.

Gupta, Charu. 2008. "(MIS) Representing the Dalit Woman: Reification of Caste and Gender Stereotypes in the Hindi Didactic Literature of Colonial India." *Indian Historical Review* 35 (2):101–124.

Gupta, Divya. 2011. "Inside India's Surrogacy Industry." *Guardian*, http://www.the-guardian.com/world/2011/dec/06/surrogate-mothers-india.

Gupta, Jyotsna Agnihotri. 2006. "Towards Transnational Feminisms: Some Reflections and Concerns in Relation to the Globalization of Reproductive Technologies." *European Journal of Women's Studies* 13 (1):23–38.

———. 2012. "Reproductive Biocrossings: Indian Egg Donors and Surrogates in the Globalized Fertility Market." *International Journal of Feminist Approaches to Bioethics* 5 (1):25–51.

Haimowitz, Rebecca, and Vaishali Sinha, dirs. 2010. *Made in India*. Brooklyn and San Francisco: Chicken and Egg Pictures. DVD.

Halliburton, Murphy. 2009. *Mudpacks and Prozac: Experiencing Ayurvedic, Biomedical and Religious Healing*. Walnut Creek: Left Coast Press.

Hamdy, Sherine. 2012. *Our Bodies Belong to God : Organ Transplants, Islam, and the Struggle for Human Dignity in Egypt*. Berkeley: University of California Press.

Hamilton, Brady E., Joyce A. Martin, and Stephanie J. Ventura. 2013. "Births: Preliminary Data for 2012." *National Vital Statistics Reports* 62 (3):1–20.

Hammerstad, Kathrine, and Marthe Haugdal. 2010. "Nordmenn på «babyshopping»-toppen i Europa" (Norwegians Top the List of Baby-Shoppers in Europe). *VG Nett*, http://www.vg.no/helse/artikkel.php?artid=591934.

Han, Sallie. 2013. *Pregnancy in Practice: Expectation and Experience in the Contemporary U.S.* New York: Berghahn Books.

Harding, Sandra. 1991. *Whose Science, Whose Knowledge?* Ithaca: Cornell University Press.

Harrison, Laura. 2014. "'I Am the Baby's Real Mother': Reproductive Tourism, Race, and the Transnational Construction of Kinship." *Women's Studies International Forum* 47:145–156.

Haworth, Abigail. 2007. "Surrogate Mothers: Womb for Rent." *Marie Claire, http://www.marieclaire.com/politics/news/a638/surrogate-mothers-india/.*

Hegde, Radha S. 1999. "Sons and (M)others: Framing the Maternal Body and the Politics of Repoduction in a South Indian Context." *Women's Studies in Communication* 22 (1):25–44.

Hoang, Kimberly Kay. 2015. *Dealing in Desire: Asian Ascendancy, Western Decline, and the Hidden Currencies of Global Sex Work*. Berkeley: University of California Press.

Hochschild, Arlie Russell. 1983. *The Managed Heart: Commercialization of Human Feeling*. Berkeley: University of California Press.

———. 2009. "Childbirth at the Global Crossroads." *American Prospect*, http://prospect.org/article/childbirth-global-crossroads-0.

———. 2012. *Outsourced Self: Intimate Life in Market Times.* New York: Metropolitan Books.

Hodges, Sarah. 2006. *Reproductive Health in India: History, Politics, Controversies.* New Delhi: Orient Longman.

Hopkins, Kristine. 2000. "Are Brazilian Women Really Choosing to Deliver by Cesarean?" *Social Science & Medicine* 51 (5):725–740.

Howell, Signe. 2006. *The Kinning of Foreigners: Transnational Adoption in a Global Perspective.* New York: Berghahn Books.

Howell, Signe, and Marit Melhuus. 2007. "Race, Biology and Culture in Contemporary Norway: Identity and Belonging in Adoption, Donor Gametes and Immigration." In *Race, Ethnicity and Nation: Perspectives from Kinship and Genetics,* edited by Peter Wade, 53–71. New York: Berghahn Books.

IANS. 2008. "Surrogacy a $445 Million Business in India." *India Today,* http://indiatoday.intoday.in/story/'Surrogacy+a+$445+mn+business+in+India'/1/13810.html.

IIPS. 2007. *National Family Health Survey (NFHS-3), 2005–06: India: Volume 1.* Mumbai: International Institute for Population Sciences.

Ikemoto, Lisa C. 2009. "Reproductive Tourism: Equality Concerns in the Global Market for Fertility Services." *Law and Inequality: A Journal of Theory and Practice* 27:277–309.

India Today. 2009. "Surrogate Babies Born in India Are Indians." http://indiatoday.intoday.in/site/Story/70679/India/'Surrogate+babies+born+in+India+are+Indians'.html?page=0.

Indian Council of Medical Research. 2000. *Ethical Guidelines for Biomedical Research on Human Subjects.* New Delhi: Indian Council of Medical Research.

Inhorn, Marcia C. 1994. *Quest for Conception: Gender, Infertility, and Egyptian Medical Traditions.* Philadelphia: University of Pennsylvania Press.

———. 2004. "Privacy, Privatization, and the Politics of Patronage: Ethnographic Challenges to Penetrating the Secret World of Middle Eastern, Hospital-Based In Vitro Fertilization." *Social Science & Medicine* 59 (10):2095–2108.

———. 2011. "Globalization and Gametes: Reproductive 'Tourism,' Islamic Bioethics, and Middle Eastern Modernity." *Anthropology & Medicine* 18 (1):87–103. doi: 10.1080/13648470.2010.525876.

———. 2015. *Cosmopolitan Conceptions: IVF Sojourns in Global Dubai.* Durham: Duke University Press.

Inhorn, Marcia C., and Pasquale Patrizio. 2009. "Rethinking Reproductive 'Tourism' as Reproductive 'Exile.'" *Fertility and Sterility* 92 (3):904–906.

Iyer, Malathy, and Pratibha Masand. 2011. "Aishwarya Rai Effect: Not Old or Posh to Push for Natural Delivery." *Times of India,* November 18.

Jain, Simmi. 2003. *Encyclopaedia of Indian Women through the Ages: Period of Freedom Struggle.* Delhi: Gyan Publishing House.

Jaisinghani, Bella. 2010. "Maid-to-Order Surrogate Mums." *Times of India,* http://timesofindia.indiatimes.com/articleshow/5783263.cms.

Janwalkar, Mayura. 2012. "17-Yr-Old Egg Donor Dead, HC Questions Fertility Center's Role." *Indian Express,* http://archive.indianexpress.com/news/17yrold-egg-donor-dead-hc-questions-fertility-centres-role/973327/0.

Janzen, John. 1978. *The Quest for Therapy: Medical Pluralism in Lower Zaire*. Berkeley: University of California Press.

Jeffery, Patricia, Roger Jeffery, and Andrew Lyon. 1989. *Labour Pains and Labour Power: Women and Childbearing in India*. London: Zed Books.

Johnson, Christopher H., Bernhard Jussen, David Warren Sabean, and Simon Teuscher. 2013. *Blood and Kinship: Matter for Metaphor from Ancient Rome to the Present*. Oxford: Berghahn Books.

Jolly, Margaret, and Kalpana Ram. 2001. *Borders of Being: Citizenship, Fertility, and Sexuality in Asia and the Pacific*. Ann Arbor: University of Michigan Press.

Jones, O. Hunter. 1976. "Cesarean Section in Present-Day Obstetrics. Presidential Address." *American Journal of Obstetrics and Gynecology* 126 (5):521–530.

Jordan, Brigitte, and Robbie Davis-Floyd. 1992. *Birth in Four Cultures: A Crosscultural Investigation of Childbirth in Yucatan, Holland, Sweden, and the United States*. Prospect Heights: Waveland Press.

Jung, Moon-Kie. 2006. "Racialization in the Age of Empire: Japanese and Filipino Labor in Colonial Hawai'i." *Critical Sociology* 32 (2–3):403–424. doi: 10.1163/156916306777835321.

Kamin, Debra. 2015. "Israel Evacuates Surrogate Babies from Nepal but Leaves the Mothers Behind." *Time*, http://time.com/3838319/israel-nepal-surrogates/.

Kanaaneh, Rhoda Ann. 2000. "New Reproductive Rights and Wrongs in the Galilee." In *Conception across Cultures: Technologies, Choices, Constraints*, edited by Andrew Russell, Elisa J. Sobo, and Mary S. Thompson, 161–178. London: Berg.

———. 2002. *Birthing the Nation: Strategies of Palestinian Women in Israel*. Berkeley: University of California Press.

Kannan, Shilpa. 2009. "Regulators Eye India's Surrogacy Sector." *BBC World News*, http://news.bbc.co.uk/2/hi/business/7935768.stm.

Kashyap, Lina D. 2007. "Indian Families in Transition: Implications for Family Policy." In *The Family in the New Millenium*, edited by A. Scott Loveless and Thomas B. Holman. Westport, Conn.: Praeger Publishers.

Kashyap, Pooja. 2011. "Test-Tube Babies No Real Option in Patna." *Times of India*, http://timesofindia.indiatimes.com/city/patna/Test-tube-babies-no-real-option-in-Patna/articleshow/8210019.cms?referral=PM.

Kempadoo, Kamala. 2005. *Trafficking and Prostitution Reconsidered: New Perspectives on Migration, Sex Work, and Human Rights*. Boulder: Paradigm.

Knoche, Jonathan W. 2014. "Health Concerns and Ethical Considerations regarding International Surrogacy." *International Journal of Gynecology & Obstetrics* 126 (2):183–186.

Krishnaraj, Maithreyi. 2010. *Motherhood in India: Glorification Without Empowerment?* New Delhi: Routledge.

Kroløkke, Charlotte. 2012. "From India with Love: Troublesome Citizens of Fertility Travel." *Cultural Politics* 8 (2):307–325. doi: 10.1215/17432197–1575183.

Layne, Linda. 1999. *Transformative Motherhood: On Giving and Getting in a Consumer Culture*. New York: NYU Press.

Lee, Rachel, and Sau-Ling Cynthia Wong. 2003. *Asian America.net: Ethnicity, Nationalism, and Cyberspace*. New York: Routledge.

Lee, Richard. 1992. "Demystifying Primitive Communism." In *Civilization in Crisis*, edited by Christine Ward Gailey, 73–94. Gainesville: University Press of Florida.

Lewin, Tamar. 2014. "Surrogates and Couples Face a Maze of Laws, State by State." *New York Times*, September 18.

Lopez, Iris. 2008. *Matters of Choice: Puerto Rican Women's Struggle for Reproductive Freedom*. New Brunswick: Rutgers University Press.

Lumbiganon, Pisake, Malinee Laopaiboon, A. Metin Gülmezoglu, João Paulo Souza, Surasak Taneepanichskul, Pang Ruyan, Deepika Eranjanie Attygalle, Naveen Shrestha, Rintaro Mori, and Nguyen Duc Hinh. 2010. "Method of Delivery and Pregnancy Outcomes in Asia: The WHO Global Survey on Maternal and Perinatal Health 2007–08." *Lancet* 375 (9713):490–499.

Lynch, Caitrin. 2007. *Juki Girls, Good Girls: Gender and Cultural Politics in Sri Lanka's Global Garment Industry*. Ithaca: Cornell University Press.

Mahapatra, Dhananjay. 2008. "Baby Manji's Case Throws Up Need for Law on Surrogacy." *Times of India*, http://timesofindia.indiatimes.com/NEWS/India/Baby-Manjis-case-throws-up-need-for-law-on-surrogacy/articleshow/3400842.cms.

Mahmood, Saba. 2005. *Politics of Piety: The Islamic Revival and the Feminist Subject*. Princeton: Princeton University Press.

Majumdar, Anindita. 2013. "Transnational Surrogacy: The 'Public' Selection of Selective Discourse." *Economic and Political Weekly* 48 (45–46):24–27.

———. 2014. "Nurturing an Alien Pregnancy: Surrogate Mothers, Intended Parents and Disembodied Relationships." *Indian Journal of Gender Studies* 21 (2):199–224.

Malhotra, Aditi, and Joanna Sugden. 2015. "India's Surrogacy Industry Needs Regulation, Not a Ban, Say Women's Rights Groups." *Wall Street Journal*, http://blogs.wsj.com/indiarealtime/2015/11/17/indias-surrogacy-industry-needs-regulation-not-a-ban-say-womens-rights-groups/.

Mamo, Laura. 2007. *Queering Reproduction: Achieving Pregnancy in the Age of Technoscience*. Durham: Duke University Press.

Marcus, George E. 1995. "Ethnography in/of the World System: The Emergence of Multi-Sited Ethnography." *Annual Review of Anthropology* 24:95–117.

Markens, Susan. 2007. *Surrogate Motherhood and the Politics of Reproduction*. Berkeley: University of California Press.

———. 2012. "The Global Reproductive Health Market: U.S. Media Framings and Public Discourses about Transnational Surrogacy." *Social Science & Medicine* 74 (11):1745–1753. doi: 10.1016/j.socscimed.2011.09.013.

Marriott, McKim. 1976. *Hindu Transactions: Diversity without Dualism*. Chicago: University of Chicago Press.

Martin, Joyce A., Brady E. Hamilton, Paul D. Sutton, Stephanie J. Ventura, Fay Menacker, and Martha L. Munson. 2003. "Births: Final Data for 2002." *National Vital Statistics Reports* 52 (10):1–114.

Maternowska, M. Catherine. 2000. "A Clinic in Conflict: A Political Economy Case Study of Family Planning in Haiti." In *Contraception across Cultures: Technologies, Choices, Constraints*, edited by Andrew Russell, Elisa J. Sobo, and Mary S. Thompson, 103–126. Oxford: Berg.

Matorras, Roberto. 2005. "Reproductive Exile versus Reproductive Tourism." *Human Reproduction* 20 (12):3571.

Mazzaschi, Andrew, and Emily Anne McDonald. 2010. *Comparative Perspectives Symposium: Gender and Medical Tourism*. Chicago: University of Chicago Press.

McCormack, Karen. 2005. "Stratified Reproduction and Poor Women's Resistance." *Gender and Society* 19 (5):660–679.

Miles, Robert. 1989. *Racism*. London: Routledge.

Miller, Barbara. 2013. "Surrogacy Secrets." *ABC News*, http://www.abc.net.au/pm/content/2013/s3674388.htm.

Ministry of Health and Family Welfare, Government of India, New Delhi. 2000. *National Population Policy, 2000*, edited by MOHFW, Department of Family Welfare. New Delhi: Ministry of Health & Family Welfare.

Ministry of Health and Family Welfare, Government of India, Indian Council of Medical Research. 2005. *National Guidelines for Accreditation, Supervision and Regulation of ART Clinics in India*. New Delhi: Ministry of Health & Family Welfare and Indian Council of Medical Research.

———. 2008. *The Assisted Reproductive Technology (Regulation) Bill & Rules-2008*. New Delhi: Ministry of Health & Family Welfare and Indian Council of Medical Research.

———. 2010. *The Assisted Reproductive Technologies (Regulation) Bill & Rules-2010*. New Delhi: Ministry of Health & Family Welfare and Indian Council of Medical Research.

Mishra, U. S., and Mala Ramanathan. 2002. "Delivery-Related Complications and Determinants of Caesarean Section Rates in India." *Health Policy and Planning* 17 (1):90–98.

Mohanty, Chandra T. 1988. "Under Western Eyes: Feminist Scholarship and Colonial Discourses." *Feminist Review* 30:61–88.

Moise, J., A. Laor, Y. Armon, I. Gur, and R. Gale. 1998. "The Outcome of Twin Pregnancies after IVF." *Human Reproduction* 13 (6):1702–1705.

Mullings, Leith. 1995. "Households Headed by Women: The Politics of Race, Class, and Gender." In *Conceiving the New World Order: The Global Politics of Reproduction*, edited by Faye Ginsburg and Rayna Rapp, 122–139. Berkeley: University of California Press.

———. 1997. *On Our Own Terms: Race, Class and Gender in the Lives of African American Women*. New York: Routledge.

———. 2005. "Resistance and Resilience: The Sojourner Syndrome and the Social Context of Reproduction in Cenral Garlem." *Transforming Anthropology* 13 (2):79–91.

Mullings, Leith, and Alaka Wali. 2001. *Stress and Resilience: The Social Context of Reproduction in Central Harlem*. New York: Kluwer Academic/Plenum Publishing.

Mutryn, Cynthia S. 1993. "Psychosocial Impact of Cesarean Section on the Family: A Literature Review." *Social Science & Medicine* 37 (10):1271–1281.

Nahman, Michal. 2008. "Nodes of Desire: Romanian Egg Sellers, 'Dignity' and Feminist Alliances in Transnational Ova Exchanges." *European Journal of Women's Studies* 15 (2):65–82.

Nandy, Ashis. 1976. "Woman versus Womanliness in India: An Essay in Social and Political Psychology." *Psychoanalytic Review* 63 (2):301–315.

Naraindas, Harish, and Cristiana Bastos. 2011. "Healing Holidays? Itinerant Patients, Therapeutic Locales and the Quest for Health." *Anthropology & Medicine* 18 (1):1–6. doi: 10.1080/13648470.2010.525871.

NewsCore. 2012. "London Sperm Bank under Investigation after Couple Has Baby from Different Race." *FoxNews.com*, http://www.foxnews.com/world/2012/04/29/london-sperm-bank-under-investigation-after-couple-has-baby-from-different-race/.

Omi, Michael, and Howard Winant. 1986. *Racial Formation in the United States: From the 1960s to the 1980s, Critical Social Thought*. New York: Routledge & Kegan Paul.

———. 2015. *Racial Formation in the United States*. 3rd ed. New York: Routledge.

Ong, Aihwa. 1999. *Flexible Citizenship: The Cultural Logics of Transnationality*. Durham: Duke University Press.

Oommen, T. K. 2002. "Race, Religion, and Caste: Anthropological and Sociological Perspectives." *Comparative Sociology* 1 (2):115–126.

———. 2005. *Crisis and Contention in Indian Society*. New Delhi: Sage.

Ortiz, Ana Teresa, and Laura Briggs. 2003. "The Culture of Poverty, Crack Babies, and Welfare Cheats: The Making of the 'Healthy White Baby Crisis.'" *Social Text* 21 (3):39–57.

Outlook India. 2009. "Only Ethics Can Prevent This Cloning, There's No Law Yet." http://www.outlookindia.com/article.aspx?239759.

Pai, M., P. Sundaram, K. K. Radhakrishnan, K. Thomas, and J. P. Muliyil. 1999. "A High Rate of Caesarean Sections in an Affluent Section of Chennai: Is It Cause for Concern?" *National Medical Journal of India* 12 (4):156–158.

Pande, Amrita. 2009a. "'It May Be Her Eggs But It's My Blood': Surrogates and Everyday Forms of Kinship in India." *Qualitative Sociology* 32 (4):379–397.

———. 2009b. "Not an 'Angel,' Not a 'Whore': Surrogates as 'Dirty' Workers in India." *Indian Journal of Gender Studies* 16 (2):141–173.

———. 2010. "Commercial Surrogacy in India: Manufacturing a Perfect Mother-Worker." *Signs: Journal of Women in Culture and Society* 35 (4):969–992.

———. 2011. "Transnational Commercial Surrogacy in India: Gifts for Global Sisters?" *Reproductive BioMedicine Online* 23 (5):618–625. doi: 10.1016/j.rbmo.2011.07.007.

———. 2014a. "The Power of Narratives: Negotiating Commercial Surrogacy in India." In *Globalization and Transnational Surrogacy in India: Outsourcing Life*, edited by Sayantani DasGupta and Shamita Das Dasgupta, 87–106. Lanham, Md.: Lexington Books.

———. 2014b. "This Birth and That: Surrogacy and Stratified Motherhood in India." *philoSOPHIA* 4 (1):50–64.

———. 2014c. *Wombs in Labor: Transnational Commercial Surrogacy in India*. New York: Columbia University Press.

Pandey, Gyanendra. 1993. "Which of Us Are Hindus?" In *Hindus and Others: The Question of Identity in India Today*, edited by Gyanendra Pandey, 238–272. New Delhi: Viking.

Papreen, Nahar, et al. 2000. "Living with Infertility: Experiences among Urban Slum Populations in Bangladesh." *Reproductive Health Matters* 8 (15):33–44.

Parreñas, Rhacel Salazar. 2001. *Servants of Globalization: Women, Migration, and Domestic Work*. Stanford: Stanford University Press.

———. 2008. *The Force of Domesticity: Filipina Migrants and Domesticity*. New York: NYU Press.

———. 2011. *Illicit Flirtations: Labor, Migration, and Sex Trafficking in Tokyo*. Stanford: Stanford University Press.

Parreñas, Rhacel Salazar, Hung Cam Thai, and Rachel Silvey. 2016. "Intimate Industries: Restructuring (Im)Material Labor in Asia." *positions: asia critique* 24 (1):1–15.

Patton, Sandra. 2000. *Birth Marks: Transracial Adoption in Contemporary America*. New York: NYU Press.

Petchesky, Rosalind, and Karen Judd. 1998. *Negotiating Reproductive Rights: Women's Perspectives across Countries and Cultures*. London: Zed Books.

Phillip, Abby. 2015. "A Shocking Scandal Led Thailand to Ban Surrogacy for Hire." *Washington Post*, http://www.washingtonpost.com/blogs/worldviews/wp/2015/02/20/a-shocking-scandal-led-thailand-to-ban-commercial-surrogacy-for-hire/.

Points, Kari. 2009. "Commercial Surrogacy and Fertility Tourism in India: The Case of Baby Manji." Durham: Kenan Institute for Ethics, Duke University.

Pollock, Anne. 2003. "Complicating Power in High-Tech Reproduction: Narratives of Anonymous Paid Egg Donors." *Journal of Medical Humanities* 24 (3–4):241–263.

Potter, Joseph E., Elza Berquó, Ignez H. O. Perpétuo, Ondina Fachel Leal, Kristine Hopkins, Marta Rovery Souza, and Maria Célia de Carvalho Formiga. 2001. "Unwanted Caesarean Sections among Public and Private Patients in Brazil: Prospective Study." *British Medical Journal* 323 (7322):1155–1158.

Prakash, Satya. 2010. "Surrogacy Not for Married Couples Only: Draft Law." *Hindustan Times*, http://www.hindustantimes.com/News-Feed/India/Surrogacy-not-for-married-couples-only-Draft-law/Article1–560762.aspx.

Puri, Chander P., Indira Hinduja, and Kusum Zaveri. 2000. "Need and Feasibility of Providing Assisted Reproductive Technologies for Infertility Management in Resource-Poor Settings." *ICMR Bulletin* 30 (6–7):55–62.

Qadeer, Imrana. 2002. "Primary Health Care: From Adjustment to Reform." In *Reforming India's Social Sector Poverty, Nutrition, Health, and Education*, edited by K. Seeta Prabhu and R. Sudarshan. New Delhi: Social Science Press.

———. 2010. "New Reproductive Technologies and India's Transitional Health System." In *Making Babies: Birth Markets and Assisted Reproductive Technologies in India*, edited by Sandhya Srinivasan, 1–21. New Delhi: Zubaan.

Quiroga, Seline Szkupinski. 2007. "Blood Is Thicker than Water: Policing Donor Insemination and the Reproduction of Whiteness." *Hypatia* 22 (2):141–160.

Ragoné, Helena. 1994. *Surrogate Motherhood: Conception in the Heart.* Boulder: Westview Press.

———. 1996. "Chasing the Blood Tie: Surrogate Mothers, Adoptive Mothers and Fathers." *American Ethnologist* 23 (2):352–365.

———. 1998. "Incontestable Motivations." In *Reproducing Reproduction: Kinship, Power, and Technological Innovation,* edited by Sarah Franklin and Helena Ragoné, 118–131. Philadelphia: University of Pennsylvania Press.

Ragoné, Helena, and France Widdance Twine. 2000. *Ideologies and Technologies of Motherhood: Race, Class, Sexuality, Nationalism.* New York: Routledge.

Rai, Saritha. 2010. "More and More Indians Want Egg Donors, but Only If They're from the Right Caste." *MinnPost,* http://www.minnpost.com/global-post/2010/09/more-and-more-indians-want-egg-donors-only-if-theyre-right-caste.

Rajadhyaksha, Madhavi. 2013. "No Surrogacy Visa for Gay Foreigners." *Times of India,* http://timesofindia.indiatimes.com/india/No-surrogacy-visa-for-gay-foreigners/articleshow/18066771.cms.

Ramasubban, Radhika, and Shireen Jejeebhoy. 2000. *Women's Reproductive Health in India.* Jaipur: Rawat Publications.

Rapp, Rayna. 2001. "Gender, Body, Biomedicine: How Some Feminist Concerns Dragged Reproduction to the Center of Social Theory." *Medical Anthropology Quarterly* 15 (4):466–477.

———. 2011. "Reproductive Entanglements: Body, State and Culture in the Dys/regulation of Childbearing." *Social Research* 78 (3):693–718.

Raymond, Janice G. 1993. *Women as Wombs: Reproductive Technologies and the Battle over Women's Freedom.* San Francisco: HarperSanFrancisco.

Riggs, Damien W., and Clemence Due. 2012. "Representations of Surrogacy in Submissions to a Parliamentary Inquiry in New South Wales." *Techné: Research in Philosophy and Technology* 16 (1):71–84.

Roberts, Dorothy. 1997. *Killing the Black Body: Race, Reproduction and the Meaning of Liberty.* New York: Pantheon Books.

———. 2002. *Shattered Bonds: The Color of Child Welfare.* New York: Basic Books.

———. 2009. "Race, Gender, and Genetic Technologies: A New Reproductive Dystopia?" *Signs* 34 (4):783–804.

Roberts, Elizabeth F. S. 2012. *God's Laboratory: Assisted Reproduction in the Andes.* Berkeley: University of California Press.

Roberts, Elizabeth F. S., and Nancy Scheper-Hughes. 2011. "Introduction: Medical Migrations." *Body & Society* 17 (2–3):1–30.

Rothman, Barbara Katz. 1988. "Reproductive Technology and the Commodification of Life." In *Embryos, Ethics, and Women's Rights,* edited by Elaine Baruch, Amadeo D'Adamo, and Joni Seager, 95–100. New York: Haworth Press.

———. 1989. *Recreating Motherhood.* New York: Norton.

Roy, Sandip. 2013. "Surrogacy and Homophobia: India Bans Gay Parents." *First Post*, http://www.firstpost.com/living/surrogacy-and-homophobia-india-bans-gay-parents-596203.html.

Roy, Somnath. 1985. "Primary Health Care in India." *Health and Population—Perspectives and Issues* 8 (3):135–167.

Roy, Sumitra Deb. 2010a. "Bar Our Nationals, European Countries Tell Surrogacy Clinics." *Times of India*, http://articles.timesofindia.indiatimes.com/2010–07–14/india/28305352_1_surrogacy-clinics-citizenship-rights.

———. 2010b. "French Gay Dad May Lose Surrogate Kids." *Times of India*, http://articles.timesofindia.indiatimes.com/2010–06–09/india/28304803_1_gay-father-surrogate-kids-surrogacy.

———. 2011. "Stateless Twins Live in Limbo." *Times of India*, http://articles.timesofindia.indiatimes.com/2011–02–02/mumbai/28374760_1_fertility-clinic-twins-crime-branch.

Rudrappa, Sharmila. 2010. "Making India the 'Mother Destination': Outsourcing Labor to Indian Surrogates." *Research in the Sociology of Work* 20:253–285.

———. 2012. "Working India's Reproductive Assembly Line: Surrogacy and Reproductive Rights?" *Western Humanities Review* Fall:77–101.

———. 2014. "Mother India: Outsourcing Labor to Indian Surrogates." In *Globalization and Transnational Surrogacy in India: Outsourcing Life*, edited by Sayantani DasGupta and Shamita Das DasGupta, 240–271. New York: Lexington Books.

———. 2015. *Discounted Life: The Price of Global Surrogacy in India*. New York: NYU Press.

Said, Edward. 1978. *Orientalism*. New York: Vintage.

Sama. 2010. "Critique of the Draft Assisted Reproductive Technologies (Regulation) Bill & Rules-2008." In *Making Babies: Birth Markets and Assisted Reproductive Technologies in India*, edited by Sandhya Srinivasan, 126–138. New Delhi: Zubaan.

———. 2011. "The Regulation of Surrogacy in India: Questions and Complexities." In *Sama-Resource Group for Women and Health*. New Delhi: Sama-Resource Group for Women and Health.

Sangari, Kumkum, and Sudesh Vaid. 1989. "Recasting Women: An Introduction." In *Recasting Women: Essays in Indian Colonial History*, edited by Kumkum Sangari and Sudesh Vaid, 1–26. New Brunswick: Rutgers University Press.

Sarojini, N. B., and Aastha Sharma. 2009. "The Draft ART (Regulation) Bill: In Whose Interest?" *Indian Journal of Medical Ethics* 6 (1):36–37.

Schieve, Laura A., Susan F. Meikle, Cynthia Ferre, Herbert B. Peterson, Gary Jeng, and Lynne S. Wilcox. 2002. "Low and Very Low Birth Weight in Infants Conceived with Use of Assisted Reproductive Technology." *New England Journal of Medicine* 346 (10):731–737.

Schneider, David. 1969. "Kinship, Nationality and Religion in American Culture: Toward a Definition of Kinship." In *Forms of Symbolic Action*, edited by Victor Turner, 116–125. New Orleans: American Ethnological Society.

———. 1980. *American Kinship: A Cultural Account*. Chicago: Umiversity of Chicago Press.

Schulz, Sandra. 2008. "The Life Factory: In India, Surrogacy Has Become a Global Business." *Der Spiegel Online*, http://www.spiegel.de/international/world/the-life-factory-in-india-surrogacy-has-become-a-global-business-a-580209.html.

Shaffer, Ellen R., and Joseph E. Brenner. 2004. "International Trade Agreements: Hazards to Health?" *International Journal of Health Services* 34 (3):467–481.

Shankar, Ramesh. 2015. Govt Bans Commercial Surrogacy in India. *Pharmabiz.com*, http://www.pharmabiz.com/NewsDetails.aspx?aid=91582&sid=1.

Sharma, Surabhi, dir. 2012. *Can We See the Baby Bump, Please?* New Delhi: Sama-Resource Group for Women and Health.

Sheth, Falguni A. 2009. *Toward a Political Philosophy of Race*. Albany: SUNY Press.

Shetty, Priya. 2012. "India's Unregulated Surrogacy Industry." *Lancet* 380 (9854):1633–1634. doi: 10.1016/S0140-6736(12)61933-3.

Sinha, Indrani, and Shamita Das Dasgupta. 2009. *Mothers for Sale: Women in Kolkata's Sex Trade*. Kolkata, India: Dasgupta Alliance.

Sinha, Kounteya. 2011. "Indians' Growing Healthcare Expenses Concern WHO." *Times of India*, http://articles.timesofindia.indiatimes.com/2011-11-02/india/30349668_1_drug-procurement-therapeutics-committee-medicines.

Sinha, Mrinalini. 2000. "Refashioning Mother India: Feminism and Nationalism in Late-Colonial India." *Feminist Studies* 26 (3):623–644.

———. 2006. *Specters of Mother India: The Global Restructuring of an Empire*. Durham: Duke University Press.

Sloan, Kathleen, and Jennifer Lahl. 2014. "Inconvenient Truths about Commercial Surrogacy." *Twin Cities*, http://www.twincities.com/columnists/ci_25470963/sloan-lahl-inconvenient-truths-about-commercial-surrogacy.

Smith, Carol A. 1997. "The Symbolics of Blood: Mestizaje in the Americas." *Identities* 3 (4):495–521.

Speert, Harold. 1980. *Obstetrics and Gynecology in America: A History*. Baltimore: Waverly Press.

Spivak, Gayatri Chakravorty. 1988. "Can the Subaltern Speak?" In *Marxism and the Interpretation of Culture*, edited by Cary Nelson and Lawrence Grossberg. London: Macmillan.

Stoler, Ann Laura. 1995. *Race and the Education of Desire: Foucault's "History of Sexuality" and the Colonial Order of Things*. Durham: Duke University Press.

Strathern, Marilyn. 1992. *Reproducing the Future: Essays on Anthropology, Kinship and the New Reproductive Technologies*. New York: Routledge.

———. 2012. "Gifts Money Cannot Buy." *Social Anthropology* 20 (4):397–410. doi: 10.1111/j.1469-8676.2012.00224.x.

Subramanian, S. V., Leland K. Ackerson, Malavika Subramanyam, and Kavita Sivaramakrishnan. 2008. "Health Inequalities in India: The Axes of Stratification." *Brown Journal of World Affairs* 14 (2):127–138.

Sullivan, Elizabeth A., Michael G. Chapman, Yueping A. Wang, and G. David Adamson. 2010. "Population-Based Study of Cesarean Section after In Vitro Fertilization in Australia." *Birth* 37 (3):184–191.

Sundari Ravindran, T. K., and P. Balasubramanian. 2004. "'Yes' to Abortion but 'No' to Sexual Rights: The Paradoxical Reality of Married Women in Rural Tamil Nadu, India." *Reproductive Health Matters* 12 (23):88–99.

Taffel, Selma M., Paul J. Placek, and Teri Liss. 1987. "Trends in the United States Cesarean Section Rate and Reasons for the 1980–85 Rise." *American Journal of Public Health* 77 (8):955–959.

Taussig, Karen-Sue, Rayna Rapp, and Deborah Heath. 2008. "Flexible Eugenics: Technologies of the Self in the Age of Genetics." *Anthropologies of Modernity: Foucault, Governmentality, and Life Politics*: 194–212.

Teman, Elly. 2008. "The Social Construction of Surrogacy Research: An Anthropological Critique of the Psychosocial Scholarship on Surrogate Motherhood." *Social Science & Medicine* 67 (7):1104–1112.

———. 2010. *Birthing a Mother: The Surrogate Body and the Pregnant Self*. Berkeley: University of California Press.

Tewary, Amarnath. 2012. "At a Sperm Bank in Bihar, Caste Divisions Start before Birth." *New York Times*, http://india.blogs.nytimes.com/2012/07/12/at-a-sperm-bank-in-bihar-caste-divisions-start-before-birth/.

Thompson, Charis. 2001. "Strategic Naturalizing: Kinship in an Infertility Clinic." In *Relative Values: Reconfiguring Kinship Studies*, edited by Sarah Franklin and Susan McKinnon, 175–202. Durham: Duke University Press.

———. 2005. *Making Parents: The Ontological Choreography of Reproductive Technologies*. Cambridge: MIT Press.

———. 2006. "Race Science." *Theory, Culture & Society* 23 (2–3):547–549. doi: 10.1177/0263276406023002100.

———. 2009. "Skin Tone and the Persistence of Biological Race in Egg Donation for Assisted Reproduction." In *Shades of Difference: Why Skin Color Matters*, edited by Evelyn Nakano Glenn. Stanford: Stanford University Press.

———. 2011. "Medical Migrations Afterword: Science as a Vacation?" *Body & Society* 17 (2–3):205–213.

Times of India. 2012a. "Surrogate Mother Dies of Complications." http://timesofindia.indiatimes.com/city/ahmedabad/Surrogate-mother-dies-of-complications/articleshow/13181592.cms.

———. 2012b. "U.S. Woman Advised to Bring Husband or Adopt Surrogate Baby." http://articles.timesofindia.indiatimes.com/2012-01-29/hyderabad/30675754_1_tatkal-scheme-passport-officer-surrogate-baby.

Tinker, Hugh. 1954. *The Foundations of Local Self-Government in India, Pakistan and Burma*. London: Pall Mall Press.

Twine, France Widdance. 2011. *Outsourcing the Womb: Race, Class, and Gestational Surrogacy in a Global Market*. New York: Routledge.

Vaid, Jyotsna. 2009. "Fair Enough? Color and the Commodification of Self in Indian Matrimonials." In *Shades of Difference: Why Skin Color Matters*, edited by Evelyn Nakano Glenn, 148–165. Stanford: Stanford University Press.

Van Hollen, Cecilia. 2003a. *Birth on the Threshold: Childbirth and Modernity in South Asia*. Berkeley: University of California Press.

———. 2003b. "Invoking Vali: Painful Technologies of Modern Birth in South India." *Medical Anthropology Quarterly* 17 (1):49–77.

———. 2013. *Birth in the Age of AIDS: Women, Reproduction, and HIV/AIDS in India*. Stanford: Stanford University Press.

Venkataratnam, Rajagopalan. 1973. *Medical Sociology in an Indian Setting*. New Delhi: Macmillan.

———. 1987. "Health System and the Polity: A Note on Indian Scene." In *Medical Care: Readings in Medical Sociology*, edited by Sheo Kumar Lal and Ambika Chandani, 16–27. New Delhi: Jainsons Publications.

Villar, José, Guillermo Carroli, Nelly Zavaleta, Allan Donner, Daniel Wojdyla, Anibal Faundes, Alejandro Velazco, Vicente Bataglia, Ana Langer, and Alberto Narváez. 2007. "Maternal and Neonatal Individual Risks and Benefits Associated with Caesarean Delivery: Multicentre Prospective Study." *British Medical Journal* 335 (7628):1025.

Villar, José, Aris T. Papageorghiou, Ruyan Pang, Eric O. Ohuma, Leila Cheikh Ismail, Fernando C. Barros, Ann Lambert, Maria Carvalho, Yasmin A. Jaffer, Enrico Bertino, Michael G. Gravett, Doug G. Altman, Manorama Purwar, Ihunnaya O. Frederick, Julia A. Noble, Cesar G. Victora, Zulfiqar A. Bhutta, and Stephen H. Kennedy. 2014. "The Likeness of Fetal Growth and Newborn Size across Non-Isolated Populations in the INTERGROWTH-21st Project: The Fetal Growth Longitudinal Study and Newborn Cross-Sectional Study." *Lancet Diabetes & Endocrinology* 2 (10):781–792.

Vora, Kalindi. 2009. "Indian Transnational Surrogacy and the Commodification of Vital Energy." *Subjectivities* 28 (1):266–278.

———. 2015. *Life Support: Biocapital and the New History of Outsourced Labor*. Minneapolis: University of Minnesota Press.

Wade, Matt, and Conrad Walters. 2010. "Indian IVF Bill May Stop Gay Couple Surrogacy." *Sydney Morning Herald*, http://www.smh.com.au/lifestyle/life/indian-ivf-bill-may-stop-gay-couple-surrogacy-20100425-tlno.html.

Wade, Peter. 2007. "Race, Ethnicity and Nation: Perspectives from Kinship and Genetics." In *Race, Ethnicity and Nation: Perspectives from Kinship and Genetics*, edited by Peter Wade, 1–32. New York: Berghahn Books.

Wadley, Susan S. 1977. "Women and the Hindu Tradition." *Signs* 3 (1):113–125.

Waldby, Catherine. 2002. "Stem Cells, Tissue Cultures and the Production of Biovalue." *Health: An Interdisciplinary Journal for the Social Study of Health, Illness and Medicine* 6 (3):305–323.

Warner, Judith. 2008. "Outsourced Wombs." *New York Times*, http://opinionator.blogs.nytimes.com/2008/01/03/outsourced-wombs/?scp=1&sq=outsourced wombs&st=cse.

Warren, Kay B. 2012. "Troubling the Victim/Trafficker Dichotomy in Efforts to Combat Human Trafficking: The Unintended Consequences of Moralizing Labor Migration." *Indiana Journal of Global Legal Studies* 19 (1):105–120.

Weiner, Michael. 1997. "The Invention of Identity: Race and Nation in Pre-War Japan." In *The Construction of Racial Identities in China and Japan: Historical and Contemporary Perspectives*, edited by Frank Dikötter, 96–117. Honolulu: University of Hawai'i Press.

Weiss, Kenneth R. 2001. "Eggs Buy a College Education." *Los Angeles Times*, May 27.

Wendland, Claire L. 2007. "The Vanishing Mother: Cesarean Section and 'Evidence-Based Obstetrics.'" *Medical Anthropology Quarterly* 21 (2):218–233.

Whitelaw, Anna. 2012. "Hundreds Pay for Overseas Surrogacy." *Sydney Morning Herald*, http://www.smh.com.au/opinion/political-news/hundreds-pay-for-overseas-surrogacy-20120602–1zp1u.html.

Whittaker, Andrea, Lenore Manderson, and Elizabeth Cartwright. 2010. "Patients without Borders: Understanding Medical Travel." *Medical Anthropology* 29 (4):336–343.

Whittaker, Andrea, and Amy Speier. 2010. "'Cycling Overseas': Care, Commodification, and Stratification in Cross-Border Reproductive Travel." *Medical Anthropology* 29 (4):363–383.

WHO. 2012. "India: Country Cooperation Strategy." Geneva: World Health Organization.

Williams, Holly. 2013a. "Are Indian Surrogacy Programs Exploiting Impoverished Women?" *ABC News*, http://www.cbsnews.com/8301–18563_162–57579212/are-indian-surrogacy-programs-exploiting-impoverished-women/.

———. 2013b. "Baby Boom: Indian Women Giving Birth to U.S. Babies." *CBS News*, http://www.cbsnews.com/8301–18563_162–57578967/baby-boom-indian-women-giving-birth-to-u.s-babies/.

Williams, Ian, and Rory Kress. 2012. "A Baby Made in India: A Couple's Dream Comes True." *Today*, http://todayhealth.today.com/_news/2012/05/28/11883566-a-baby-made-in-india-a-couples-dream-comes-true?lite.

Winant, Howard. 2004. *The New Politics of Race: Globalism, Difference, Justice*. Minneapolis: University of Minnesota Press.

Worthington, Roger P., and Anupriya Gogne. 2011. "Cultural Aspects of Primary Healthcare in India: A Case-Based Analysis." *Asia Pacific Family Medicine* 10 (8):1–5.

Yngvesson, Barbara. 2010. *Belonging in an Adopted World: Race, Identity and Transnational Adoption*. Chicago: University of Chicago Press.

Yuval-Davis, Nira, Kalpana Kannabiran, and Ulrike M. Vieten. 2006. *The Situated Politics of Belonging*. London: Sage Publications.

Zelizer, Viviana A. 2010. *Economic Lives: How Culture Shapes the Economy*. Princeton: Princeton University Press.

INDEX

Page references followed by a t *indicate a table.*

Accreditation, Supervision & Regulation of ART Clinics in India, 45
ACS (American Citizen Services Unit), 129–30, 136
adoption: in Australia, 30, 88; humanitarian justifications for, 65; in Israel, 79; in Norway, 138; reasons for rejecting, 243n3; vs. transnational surrogacy, 73–74; in the United States, 65; waiting periods for, 88
Agarwal, Kanupriya (*pseud.* Durga), 39–40
agency and power in surrogates' lives, 195–222; agents' work, 197–99, 207–16, 220–21; Antara and Rahul's story (case study), 196, 208–16, 220–21, 225; constrained agency, 204–8; the contract process, 207–8; gender/reproductive/family relations, 201–4; marriage and gender relations, 203–4, 216–20; Nishi's story (case study), 195–96, 198, 203–8, 221, 243n4 (ch 7); overview of, 25, 195–99; Parvati and Kapil's story (case study), 196, 216–21; surrogacy likened to sex work, 219; surrogates as breeders vs. breadwinners, 199–200, 242n3
Agreement on Trade Related Intellectual Property Rights (TRIPS), 37
Ahearn, Laura, 202
Ahmed, Leila, 241n4 (ch 2)
Alma Ata declaration, 36
Althusser, Louis, 13

Ambedkar, B. R., 236–37, 243n4 (appendix)
American Citizen Services Unit (ACS), 129–30, 136
American College of Obstetricians and Gynecologists, 175
Anagnost, Ann, 65
Anderson, Benedict, 12, 127
anthropology, multisited research vs. area studies in, 16–17
Appadurai, Arjun, 11
ARTs (assisted reproductive technologies), 34, 45, 101, 161; artificial wombs, 75; in India, history of, 39–42, 45, 240n3; in Indian infertility clinics, 8, 237–38; as infertility treatment, 96; low birth weight of babies conceived by, 175; multiple pregnancies conceived by, 175; norms aligned with, 6; in Norway, 137–39; racial preferences of consumers of, 97; regulations regarding, 5–6; scope of, 5; success rates of, 161; test-tube babies, earliest, 39–40. *See also* doctors' medicalization of women's pregnancies; Indian surrogacy; IVF; surrogacy
Asians, racialization of, 150
assisted reproductive technologies. *See* ARTs
Australia: adoption in, 30, 88; cesarean rates in, 175; surrogacy laws in, 30–31, 88
Ayurvedic medicine, 75

ABOUT THE AUTHOR

Daisy Deomampo is Assistant Professor of Anthropology at Fordham University. She is a medical and cultural anthropologist whose research interests include science and technology studies, gender and critical race studies, reproduction, and global health.